Voyeurism

Simon Duff

Voyeurism

A Case Study

palgrave
macmillan

Simon Duff
University of Nottingham
Nottingham, UK

ISBN 978-3-319-97159-9 ISBN 978-3-319-97160-5 (eBook)
https://doi.org/10.1007/978-3-319-97160-5

Library of Congress Control Number: 2018950419

This Palgrave Pivot imprint is published by the registered company Springer Nature Switzerland AG
The registered company address is: Gewerbestrasse 11, 6330 Cham, Switzerland

For House and KS

Acknowledgements

My clinical colleagues have my upmost respect and admiration for the work that they do, day in and day out, and the inspiration they are to my thinking. All the wrong thoughts are entirely my own. As always, my gorgeous and talented family and friends have been appropriately distracting and given me perspective. Too much perspective.

Contents

CHAPTER 1

Introduction

Abstract The opening chapter situates the issue of voyeurism within the context of the difficulties of understanding any form of sexual offending and the importance of considering the broadest range of possible factors that may play a role in the development of sexual behaviour. It also presents the working definition of voyeurism that will be used throughout the book.

Keywords Voyeurism · Sexual offending · Frotteurism

Herein is an effort to provide consideration of behaviour and people that have variously been referred to as voyeurism (Karpman, 1954), scopophilia (Hirschfield, 1948; Rosen, 1979), inspectionalism (Colman, 1964), peepers (Gebhard, Gagnon, Pomeroy, & Christenson, 1965), and voyeurs (Smith, 1976). That there are so many names to describe the activity and the actors might suggest that there is a wealth of fact and theory which, given the correct amount of effort, would provide psychological insight into the origins, development, and treatment of the behaviour once it becomes harmful to the actor or to others. Unfortunately, this is untrue as voyeurism has not attracted the same level of attention as other kinds of sexual behaviour, whether they be benign or offending in nature. As McAnulty, Adams, and Dillon (2001) have written, "Overall, voyeurism remains one of the least studied sexual deviations" (p. 775). It is also the case that some authors have

S. Duff, *Voyeurism*, https://doi.org/10.1007/978-3-319-97160-5_1

questioned whether it is appropriate to consider voyeurism as a distinct issue given that, according to them, there are so few cases that are not accompanied by other paraphilias such as exhibitionism and frotteurism (see Langevin, Paitich, & Russon, 1985). So, partly because the space of voyeurism remains uncharted and partly because understanding this area of behaviour is important and fascinating, this project has been undertaken.

Any attempt to understand sexual behaviour is fraught with difficulties. To begin with, a large portion of sexual behaviour happens in our minds and we may have little access to the details of it and may decide that we don't wish to share it accurately, if at all. It is highly unlikely that sexual behaviour is not influenced by both biology and society; both play an important role in determining our individual psychology: what we attend to, what we value, what we are attracted to, what we are allowed to be attracted to, what is legitimate, and what is unholy. In the latter case, religion has had something to say about voyeurism, as it has about many behaviours. In Matthew 5:28, Jesus is reported to have said during the Sermon on the Mount, "but I tell you that everyone who gazes at a woman to lust after her has committed adultery with her already in his heart" (King James Version). If we consider that at least one role of religion was to exert an element of social control (Raven, 1999), then it appears that voyeurism has been considered problematic for a lengthy period of time (if something is not an issue then why develop a set of rules in order to control it?). The same rule could also be applied to pornography, strip shows, and celebrity sex tapes.

Our past experiences and the opportunities we will take advantage of in the future are intimately linked to how we understand, think, and behave. This is complicated enough without the addition of genders and sexualities. Having discussed sexual behaviour with colleagues, trainees, and clients over a number of years, I am well aware of the ease with which people can be upset by a view, or a question, or a bias. As upset as you may get, it is unintended. Ultimately, writing within an area that is, academically speaking, relatively unpopulated means that this is something of a journey of exploration, guided by what I think is interesting and important, with the aim of sharing some of the understanding that I have reached, although I will never know if that final goal has been achieved. If it is I hope it provokes people to go further and if it isn't I hope it provokes people to achieve what I haven't.

Another important issue to raise is how we are defining voyeurism for this journey. As with many terms, "voyeurism" has escaped its formal psychiatric definition, which is useful in some ways as it allows us to recognise the continuum of human behaviour rather than categories of normal and abnormal. The negative is that it can be used to describe a range of activities that are considered by someone to be unusual or negative. For example, in South Korea there is a phenomenon that in the UK we refer to as "gastronomic voyeurism", they call it "broadcast eating"; you can view, typically a young, slim woman, eating a huge meal. It is not obvious that there is any kind of sexual element and some commentators have suggested that it fulfils an important social role for single people who would otherwise dine alone, as people can interact with the eater. Viewers can also make financial donations. Voyeur is also used to describe people who spend time watching reality television, reading celebrity magazines, and focussing on other people's lives. As Levy (2015) has written, "If there was ever any doubt that we are a voyeuristic species, the fact that people want to watch these stories puts closure on this question" (p. 154). The photographer Edo Zollo has referred to his pictures as voyeuristic (www.edlondonphotography.co.uk), and as a final example, some writers have referred to "intellectual voyeurism"—"superficial and ill-informed treatment of serious ideas, apparently done for intellectual 'titillation' or to advertise, in a pretentious way, the 'sophistication' of the writer" (Leiter, 1992, p. 80).

For our purposes, what makes a behaviour or group of behaviours fit within the range of voyeurism is that it involves observation of someone or something, it is intended to be secret, and that there is some form of sexual element linked to it. In this way, behaviours that are not observational and not sexual are not included (thus, intellectual writing and watching reality television) and neither are behaviours that involve sexualised observation but are not fully secret, for example, watching strip shows or sexual live-feed videos. The latter will also disallow pornography, whether professional or amateur (e.g. celebrity sex tapes or revenge pornography where the subject(s) know that they are being filmed, even if they do not know how it might be used later), but secret pictures or recordings by a person that may be used later do fit the category of voyeurism (for example, Client A, as described by Mann, Ainsworth, Al-Attar, & Davies, 2008, who filmed women in a massage parlour and used these films for masturbation at a later date). For an early typography of digital images, it would be useful to read the work of Holmes,

Tewksbury, and Holmes (1998). It is noteworthy that some authors have suggested that it is important to differentiate between those who actively seek out opportunities to watch and those who are more opportunistic (Gebhard et al., 1965) but this is not an approach that will be taken here in part because it may be difficult to differentiate between the two because victims are unlikely to know and perpetrators may lie.

References

Coleman, J. (1964). *Abnormal psychology and modern life* (3rd ed.). Glenview, IL: Scott Foresman.

Gebhard, P. H., Gagnon, J. H., Pomeroy, W. B., & Christenson, C. V. (1965). *Sex offenders*. New York: Harper & Row.

Hirschfield, M. (1948). *Sexual anomalies and perversions*. London: Francis Alder.

Holmes, R. M., Tewksbury, R., & Holmes, S. T. (1998). Hidden JPGs: A functional alternative to voyeurism. *Journal of Popular Culture, 32*(3), 17–29.

Karpman, B. (1954). *The sexual offender and his offences*. New York, NY: Julian Press.

Langevin, R., Paitich, D., & Russon, A. E. (1985). Voyeurism: Does it predict sexual aggression or violence in general? In R. Langevin (Ed.), *Erotic preference, gender identity, and aggression in men: New research studies* (pp. 77–98). Hillsdale, NJ: Erlbaum.

Leiter, B. (1992). Intellectual voyeurism in legal scholarship. *Yale Journal of the Law and Humanities, 4*, 79–104.

Levy, M. S. (2015). *Celebrity and entertainment obsession: Understanding our addiction*. London: Rowman & Littlefield.

Mann, R. E., Ainsworth, F., Al-Attar, Z., & Davies, M. (2008). Voyeurism: Assessment and treatment. In D. R. Laws & W. T. O'Donohue (Eds.), *Sexual Deviance* (2nd ed., pp. 320–335). New York: Guilford Press.

McAnulty, R. D., Adams, H. E., & Dillon, J. (2001). Sexual deviation: Paraphilias. In P. B. Sutker & H. E. Adams (Eds.), *Comprehensive handbook of psychopathology* (3rd ed., pp. 749–773). New York, NY: Kluwer Academic.

Raven, B. H. (1999). Kurt Lewin address: Influence, power, religion, and the mechanisms of social control. *Journal of Social Issues, 55*(1), 161–186.

Rosen, I. (1979). Exhibitionism, scopophilia and voyeurism. In I. Rosen (Ed.), *Sexual deviation*. Oxford: Oxford University Press.

Smith, R. S. (1976). Voyeurism: A literature review. *Archives of Sexual Behavior, 5*(6), 585–608.

CHAPTER 2

Voyeurism in Context

Abstract This chapter considers the context for voyeurism, from the basics of how looking is important for our survival to how it is linked to sexual behaviour, and considers the complexity of identifying what voyeurism is and who might be doing it.

Keywords Attraction · Crotch-watching · Voyeurism

Our attention is captured by visual information throughout our lives for a variety of practical, automatic purposes, on a daily basis. We have all probably blinked or ducked at just the right moment to avoid being hit by a wayward cricket ball, or stepped back onto the pavement when we have noticed a motorcycle out of the corner of our eye. Visual information is crucial to our individual survival. Evolutionary psychologists tell us that it is also central to our species survival as it is used in the process of mate selection, providing at least some of the information that helps us identify sexual partners who are healthy and fertile (Fink, Hugill, & Lange, 2012; Puts et al., 2013), and this is true of both genders (Singh, 1993, 1995). In addition to these survival processes, we can consider that novelty, possible utility (what Gibson referred to as "affordances"; Gibson, 1966), and individual biases and interests can play a part in both attracting and holding our attention as we negotiate the world. Basically, people with functioning visual systems look for information and less obviously to provide information (such as, are we attending to a speaker?

S. Duff, *Voyeurism*, https://doi.org/10.1007/978-3-319-97160-5_2

[Ho, Foulsham, & Kingstone, 2015]; determining if the direction of our gaze is suggesting there is something interesting or of survival value to attend to [Mathews, Fox, Yiend, & Calder, 2003]). So, looking is not, by definition, dysfunctional or pathological; it is not necessarily indicative of anything unusual.

Similarly, that looking is linked to sexual behaviour will be of little surprise, but the complexity of it and the variability are perhaps less well known and less well understood. Sexual attraction and sexual behaviour are a mixture of perinatal and postnatal influences (Gagnon & Simon, 2005; Laws & Marshall, 1990; Woodson, 2002) and reasonably we can hypothesise that what we find visually sexually interesting may be so influenced. The body genders, body shapes, and body parts that attract us are likely to be a combination of our cognitive biases (from both nature and nurture) and social conformity, resulting in the experience that some people, some things, just are "sexy". Although it might be interesting and useful to determine if there are some shared, underlying factors that imbue sexiness to something or someone, this level of analysis has not been undertaken and may prove fruitless given the breadth of people who experience sexiness and the range of people and objects that are experienced as sexy. As such, the focus of much research in understanding the features that may result in something being identified as sexy is not so fine grained but rather is on objects, animals, people, parts of people, and people's acts.

Even at this level do we understand why we are sexually attracted to particular people? Studies have identified that symmetrical faces are more attractive (Jones, Little, Burt, & Perrett, 2004), that particular body shapes are more attractive (Swami, Jones, Einon, & Furnham, 2009), that particular smells are more attractive (Thornhill & Gangestad, 1999) but is it really the combination of these component parts that result in sexual attraction? Swami et al. (2009) found that the attractiveness of a body shape is at least partly culturally determined (although other studies do not find a cultural effect, e.g. Cunningham, Roberts, Barbee, & Druen, 1995; Langlois et al., 2000); studies have suggested that lower levels of facial symmetry might be associated with ill health, such as lung problems (Thornhill & Gangestad, 2006); smell is more attractive if the man who is smelled has a symmetrical face and the women doing the smelling are not using the contraceptive pill and are at the highest point of fertility in their menstrual cycle (Thornhill & Gangestad, 1999). Thus, even when we can identify component parts the story is far more complex than the simple addition of the components and also, as yet, the research in many areas is not consistent in its findings. Given this situation how can we hope to understand the attraction of those who are attracted to features that do not fit with social norms? Perhaps the best method is to look for those events that can act as triggers, responses to events that are unusual or catastrophic, and develop a narrative that makes sense, being mindful of Occam's razor to prevent us going too far off track and recruiting explanations that do not allow for testing and further scrutiny.

The fact that we identify people who are sexually attracted to features of the body that are less generally agreed as being sexual (that attraction is known as *partialism*) as being somewhat unusual or deviant, such as the person sexually aroused to feet, is evidence of the power of the prevailing social norms in focussing sexuality in its broadest sense to a range of shared norms. Similarly with the individual who is unable to be sexually satisfied unless their partner wears a particular pair of shoes during sex (the strict definition of *fetishism* is restricted to non-living objects). Legal systems, as expressions of social authority, also act to define how behaviour is understood and where on a continuum it lies in relation to acceptable, tolerated, and forbidden. Within this, it is also important to accept that society takes some responsibility in defining the value of some visual information. Advertising, pornography, and celebrity media expose us to images emphasising both the aspirational nature and the societal power of sexuality along with it being taboo and a valid area of public interest and scrutiny. Some of Tom Ford's campaign for their first male fragrance presented images of naked women with bottles of scent carefully placed to prevent the images being more pornographic than erotic. This is not to make any moral judgements about what is happening, that has been and continues to be covered by scholars, rather having awareness that our behaviour has to be understood within a much broader context if we are to understand it at all (Shoveller, Johnson, Langille, & Mitchell, 2004).

Another element of this context that must be appreciated is the complexity of investigating sexual behaviour beyond that particular behaviour and the physiological responses it engenders and relies on. Firstly, do adults have the introspective powers to accurately describe their thoughts and feelings related to sexual fantasy, sexual activity, and sexual feelings? If the accuracy of introspection is available, then to what extent will people honestly report, particularly if they know or suspect that their thoughts and feelings and behaviours are outside societal norms? These issues have been identified in research that has sought to understand sexual offending against children, but they remain complex (see Walton & Duff, 2017). How difficult is it to really gather data on *paedophilic* adults who do not ever offend against children because of their own concerns about the focus of their sexual attraction and an awareness that society frequently maps *paedophilia* directly onto child abuse (our current research concerned with non-offending men who are attracted to children, being investigated by Harriet Dymond, also struggles with these issues)? The issue is further compounded if we are investigating children or childhood experiences. Do children have an understanding of sexual behaviour? At what point would we define any pre-adult behaviour as experienced or performed as "sexual" in the sense that the pre-adult understands it in this way? Is it possible for an adult to provide a description of their childhood experiences without interpreting those experiences and their thoughts and feelings through the lens of their adult sexuality, adult knowledge, and adult experiences? People change, society changes and both are crucial to be mindful of in working with individuals whose behaviour currently is troubling but its roots may lie in early experiences.

Within this broader context, what do we know of behaviour that is linked to voyeurism? Studies have shown that males and females view nude images differently and, possibly, counter-intuitively. In one such study (Rupp & Wallen, 2007), males were found to spend more time, and had a higher probability of, looking at female faces whereas women who were not using contraception spent more time, and had a higher probability of, looking at male genitals. This might suggest we would expect more women to be voyeurs, given they seem to have a greater interest in viewing genitals. However, the findings may really reflect the fact that society presents naked women far more frequently than it does naked men and as such for women there is a greater novelty and curiosity to view men's genitals when the opportunity arises, as it were. It doesn't necessarily mean women are more driven to seek out opportunities to see naked men. This research fits with the self-reported fantasies and sexual behaviours of women (see Friday, 1973, 1975) which includes the elements of voyeurism including what Friday refers to as "crotch-watching". So women do engage in voyeurism, but care needs to be taken in how we interpret the relevant findings.

Recent research examining the prevalence of voyeurism in a sample of people attending to treatment for sexual behaviours supports the view that although women are voyeurs, far more men identify as, or have been identified as, voyeurs. In their sample of 3951 men and 541 women, Hopkins, Green, Carnes, and Campling (2016) found that 26 of the women were classified as voyeurs (4.8% of the sample of women). Unfortunately, the paper does not report how many men fit the voyeur criteria; they used a randomly selected sample of 214 from the total of voyeurs for statistical purposes, which is equivalent to 5.4% of the male sample. However, the total sample of voyeurs numbered 607 men (Green, personal communication, 2018), which is 15.4% of the male sample.

So we do know something of sexual looking. As suggested earlier, it informs decisions about sexual partners; we are aware of the use of sexualised images in advertisements (although research suggests that the focus can often be on the sexualised imagery rather than on the product; Simpson, Horton, & Brown, 1996), and visual pornography is aimed entirely at direct sexual stimulation, whether that leads to sexual behaviour within a relationship, solo sexual behaviour, or the possible motivation towards deviant sexual behaviours such as sexual assault or rape. Thus, much of our looking behaviour may be both sexual and entirely routine and socially acceptable. Where it isn't socially acceptable, much of it will go unnoticed because at times we do look at one another in ways that are unacceptable in particular contexts or within particular relationships, sometimes clothes slip, or we don't close a curtain or blind. Even when we do notice someone looking, the process of identifying that they are looking at us, or at anything specific, is complex. The exact direction of gaze and the focus of that gaze are hard to accurately assess for the observer. The ability to determine if something untoward is being looked at by another person, or if we are being looked at, is not trivial, as demonstrated by the studies identifying the key areas of the brain that appear sensitive to gaze (Carlin & Calder, 2013).

Sometimes, viewing that is not considered mainstream is encouraged through strip shows and personal Internet cameras, to name a few. Sometimes, we don't know we are being seen, sometimes we know we are being seen but not by whom (and don't mind, as Douglas and colleagues have suggested, is the case for some nude sunbathers; Douglas, Rasmussen, & Flanagan, 1977). The differences in prevalence between the genders described earlier raises some interesting and as yet unexplored issues. Firstly, we might wonder if, as the sample described by Hopkins et al. (2016) were attending a clinic for sexual issues, do fewer women engage in voyeurism? It is plausible that as many do but fewer identify it as a sexual problem, that fewer are caught engaging in voyeurism, or that if caught fewer are convicted or reprimanded? Perhaps we are less concerned if we are observed in private activities by women, but if that is true, why would we be less concerned?

References

Carlin, J. D., & Calder, A. J. (2013). The neural basis of eye gaze processing. *Current Opinion in Neurobiology, 23*, 450–455.

Cunningham, M. R., Roberts, A. R., Barbee, A. P., & Druen, P. B. (1995). 'Their ideas of beauty are, on the whole, the same as ours': Consistency and variability in the cross-cultural perception of female attractiveness. *Journal of Personality and Social Psychology, 68*, 261–279.

Douglas, J. D., Rasmussen, P. K., & Flanagan, C. A. (1977). *The nude beach*. Beverly Hills, CA: Sage.

Fink, B., Hugill, N., & Lange, B. P. (2012). Women's body movements are a potential cue to ovulation. *Personality and Individual Differences, 53*(6), 759–763.

Friday, N. (1973). *My Secret Garden: Women's Sexual Fantasies*. NY: Simon and Schuster.

Friday, N. (1975). *Forbidden Flowers: More Women's Sexual Fantasies*. NY: Simon and Schuster.

Gagnon, J. H., & Simon, W. (2005). *Sexual conduct: The social sources of human sexuality* (2nd ed.). New Brunswick, USA: Aldine Transaction.

Gibson, J. J. (1966). *The senses considered as perceptual systems*. Boston: Houghton Mifflin Company.

Ho, S., Foulsham, T., & Kingstone, A. (2015). Speaking and listening with the eyes: Gaze signalling during dyadic interactions. *PLoS One, 10*(8). https://doi.org/10.1371/journal.pone.0136905.

Hopkins, T. A., Green, B. A., Carnes, P. J., & Campling, S. (2016). Varieties of intrusion: Exhibitionism and voyeurism. *Sexual Addiction & Compulsivity, 23*(1), 4–33.

Jones, B. C., Little, A. C., Burt, D. M., & Perrett, D. I. (2004). When facial attractiveness is only skin deep. *Perception, 33*(5), 569–576.

Langlois, J. H., Kalakanis, L., Rubenstein, A. J., Larson, A., Hallam, M., & Smoot, M. (2000). Maxims or myths of beauty? A meta-analytic and theoretical review. *Psychological Bulletin, 126*(3), 390–423.

Laws, D. R., & Marshall, W. L. (1990). A conditioning theory of the etiology and maintenance of deviant sexual preference and behavior. In W. L. Marshall & others (eds.), *Handbook of sexual assault*. New York: Springer Science + Business Media.

Mathews, A., Fox, E., Yiend, J., & Calder, A. (2003). The face of fear: Effects of eye gaze and emotion on visual attention. *Visual Cognition, 10*(7), 823–835.

Puts, D. A., Bailey, D. H., Cárdenas, R. A., Burriss, R. P., Welling, L. L. M., Wheatley, J. R., & Dawood, K. (2013). Women's attractiveness changes with estradiol and progesterone across the ovulatory cycle. *Hormones and Behavior, 63*(1), 13–19.

Rupp, H. A., & Wallen, K. (2007). Sex differences in viewing sexual stimuli: An eye-tracking study in men and women. *Hormones and Behavior, 51*(4), 524–533.

Shoveller, J. A., Johnson, J. L., Langille, D. B., & Mitchell, T. L. (2004). Socio-cultural influences on young people's sexual behaviour. *Social Science and Medicine, 59*(3), 473–487.

Simpson, P. M., Horton, S., & Brown, G. (1996). Male nudity in advertisements: A modified replication and extension of gender and product effects. *Journal of the Academy of Marketing Science, 24*(3), 257–262.

Singh, D. (1993). Adaptive significance of female physical attractiveness: Role of waist-to-hip ratio. *Journal of Personality and Social Psychology, 65*(2), 293–307.

Singh, D. (1995). Female judgment of male attractiveness and desirability for relationships: Role of waist-to-hip ratio and financial status. *Journal of Personality and Social Psychology, 69*(6), 1089–1101.

Swami, V., Jones, J., Einon, D., & Furnham, A. (2009). Men's preferences for women's profile waist-to-hip ratio, breast size, and ethnic group in Britain and South Africa. *British Journal of Psychology, 100*, 313–325.

Thornhill, R., & Gangestad, S. W. (1999). The scent of symmetry: A human sex pheromone that signals fitness? *Evolution and Human Behavior, 20*(3), 175–201.

Thornhill, R., & Gangestad, S. W. (2006). Facial sexual dimorphism, developmental stability, and susceptibility to disease in men and women. *Evolution and Human Behavior, 27*(2), 131–144.

Walton, J. S., & Duff, S. (2017). "I'm not homosexual or heterosexual, I'm paedosexual": Exploring sexual preference for children using interpretive phenomenology. *Journal of Forensic Practice, 19*(2), 151–161.

Woodson, J. C. (2002). Including 'learned sexuality' in the organization of sexual behaviour. *Neuroscience and Biobehavioral Reviews, 26*, 69–80.

CHAPTER 3

Voyeurism

Abstract This chapter provides a summary of what we do understand about voyeurism, considering what we know about voyeurs and if their behaviour might be linked to other offending, what we know about victims and the impact of voyeurism, how the public understand voyeurism, and how society may at least support various forms of voyeuristic behaviour.

Keywords Coprophilia · Scoptophilia · Troilism · Dogging
Iconophilia

The breadth and complexity of our looking behaviour, and the subset of sexualised looking behaviour, are mostly irrelevant to the public and not yet fully scrutinised by science, and that is true for the sexualised looking behaviour that is considered both deviant and illegal, voyeurism. Voyeurism is an umbrella term concerned with the individuals who, at the extreme, require visual opportunities in order to experience sexual satisfaction, and this causes them harm or distress, and may cause harm to others. Some examples of the specific forms of voyeurism are *voyeuristic coprophilia* (viewing others defecating or urinating) and *scoptophilia* (viewing others engaging in sexual intercourse) which now, when those being viewed engage in this knowingly, is referred to in the UK as "dogging". Where someone persuades a partner to engage in sexual intercourse with a third party, whilst this third party doesn't know that

S. Duff, *Voyeurism*, https://doi.org/10.1007/978-3-319-97160-5_3

they are being observed, the behaviour is known as *troilism* (for a case example see Allen, 1969). At its most extreme, voyeurism causes distress and impairment to the voyeur, something recognised by the American Psychiatric Association (American Psychiatric Association, 2000), and to the victim(s), and at its most benign it might involve a woman coming home, finding her partner in the shower, and watching without drawing attention to her presence. Some authors have suggested that within the umbrella of voyeurism, it might be useful to think of three sub-categories (Kaplan & Krueger, 1997), namely (i) voyeurs whose sole sexual outlet is through voyeurism, (ii) voyeurs who prefer their voyeuristic behaviour but will engage in other forms of sexual behaviour, and (iii) people who only engage in voyeurism in response to some form of stress. It is likely that the psychology at the core of the different levels of voyeurism on these continua will differ and at many of these levels there will be no immediate or long-term distress to either party. However, in order to be able to manage and prevent the levels of voyeurism that do result in distress, it is important to understand voyeurism at that extreme level.

In their chapter concerned with voyeurism, Mann, Ainsworth, Al-Attar and Davies (2008) state that there is little literature concerned with the paraphilia of voyeurism and that "any research into voyeurism would be welcome" (p. 331). This aligns with the views of earlier authors: Yalom (1960) stated, "Psychiatric literature devoted to this perversion is scarce" (p. 305), and Smith (1976) wrote, "The most striking thing about the literature on voyeurism is the relative lack of material in print" (p. 585). Gebhard, Gagnon, Pomeroy, and Christenson (1965) included some attention to voyeurs in their study of sexual offending and describe the voyeur as follows:

> ...ardent fishermen, undaunted by failure and always hoping that the next time their luck will be better. Just as the fisherman will wait patiently for hours, so will the peeper wait for a female to finish some interminable minor chores before going to bed and then, like as not, she may turn off the light before undressing. Again like the fisherman who keeps a list of areas where fishing is especially good, the peeper not infrequently has in mind a number of particularly likely places to which he returns. (pp. 359–360)

Along with this rather benign description, they suggest that voyeurs tend to be the youngest child in their family, have good relationships with their parents, tend not to live in all-female homes, and are ranked high in fear of sexually transmitted diseases, amongst other features.

Since these studies and remarks, there has been some further research (e.g. Hopkins, Green, Carnes, & Campling, 2016) but for those who work clinically with these individuals, there is still little to base their assessments and interventions on. There are two reasons why knowing more about voyeurism is important: to understand more about the offenders and to understand more about the impact on victims.

Understanding the Voyeur

Yalom (1960) describes a range of voyeur clients who possess, "an exaggerated desire to see, by stealth, a member of the opposite sex in some stage of undress, in the sexual act, or in the act of excretion, which is so intense that it surpasses in importance the normal sexual act" (p. 305). Whilst some individuals simply find their interest personally troubling, for others it leads to contact with the criminal justice system. Unfortunately, in the UK it is not possible to ascertain how many individuals are arrested for voyeurism. It is an offence covered by police reporting within the category "other sexual offences", which includes everything other than rape. Although the UK Ministry of Justice overview of sexual offending in England and Wales does identify voyeuristic offences recorded by the police, they are grouped together with exposure. This is a strategy also repeated in various books that present information on voyeurism, such as the chapter by Hocken and Thorne (2012), where voyeurism and exhibitionism are grouped together. On the surface, this makes sense: one focuses on people who like to display themselves and the other on people who like to see other people. It is also perhaps telling that exhibitionists, by the nature of their offending, are more likely to be noticed and apprehended, so we know more about them, what they do, how many people do it, and how many people have had it done to them. Perhaps more subtly is the implication that these two forms of non-contact sexual offence are psychologically linked. A connection has been suggested. For example, some authors have suggested that both these behaviours, and other paraphilias, may be related as they can be expressions of obsessive–compulsive disorder. Abouesh and Clayton (1999) provide a description of an exhibitionist and a voyeur who were both treated with paroxetine and showed a decrease in their behaviour and compulsive thoughts. The fact that the same medication worked for both individuals certainly hints that there may be a link but care needs to be taken with the assumption that if one medication can treat two issues, they are necessarily related. For example, hydrocodone is used as a painkiller and as a cough suppressant.

From a psychological perspective, the official figures for voyeurism provide little scope to examine the basic demographic characteristics or the potential for increasing risk to contact offences. Some authors have sought to further our understanding by examining voyeurism through empirical studies. In studies recruiting volunteers, it is likely that only specific people volunteer to answer questions about their sexual behaviour and within that group perhaps only a subset will answer honestly (see Ahlers et al., 2011, for an example). To further complicate matters, over time and across cultures different definitions of voyeurism may be used, resulting in potential bias. For example, in their recent paper Joyal and Carpentier (2016) asked the following in order to measure the prevalence of voyeurism in a Swedish sample, "Have you ever been sexually aroused while watching a stranger, who was unaware of your presence, while they were nude, were undressing, or were having sexual relations?" Such a definition might not capture, for an individual responding, the specifics of UK law which includes a person using a lavatory (Sexual Offences Act, 2003, Section 68). Thus, any estimates of the prevalence of voyeurism may be inaccurate.

Despite these concerns, it is useful to consider the estimates that have been published in a variety of settings. Estimates from the general population suggest that voyeurism is an issue for young males, with Dawson, Bannerman and Lalumière (2016) reporting that 52% of their sample acknowledged an interest in voyeurism. In Sweden, lifetime prevalence rates for experience with voyeurism was 11.5% amongst men (Långström & Seto, 2006). More recently, Makanjuola, Adegunloye, and Adelekan (2008) found a prevalence rate of 22% for experience with paraphilic behaviours amongst 408 male and female high school teachers in Nigeria with voyeurism, the most prevalent at 10%. In Brazil, de Oliveira and Abdo (2010) found in their sample of 7022 people that 13% reported having engaged in voyeurism. In Germany, Ahlers et al. (2011) reported that 44% of a community sample of men acknowledged at least one lifetime paraphilic behaviour and the second highest was voyeurism at 18%. Considering clinical samples, Maletzky and McGovern (1991) report that in their sample of offenders treated in a sexual abuse clinic, 1.2% (60) had a primary diagnosis of voyeurism. For the sake of context, 57.3% (2865) had a primary diagnosis of heterosexual paedophilia,

15.4% (770) exhibitionism, and 0.4% (20) zoophilia. Marsh et al. (2010) estimated that 8% of a sample of 122 adult male psychiatric inpatients met the DSM-IV criteria for voyeurism. These studies suggest that voyeurism is a relatively frequent form of paraphilic behaviour. Given that Abel et al. (1987) report that their sample of 62 voyeurs claim to have engaged in 469 separate acts on average, the scale of the problem is large.

In the laboratory studies the self-rated likelihood of taking part in voyeurism is found to be higher. Examining a sample of college students ($n = 159$), 84% of men and 74% of women admitted they would engage in voyeurism if they would not get caught (Rye & Meaney, 2007). Of note is that there were no statistical differences between men and women when the voyeurism involved watching an attractive person undress; however, when it involved watching an attractive couple have sex, men were far more likely to engage in this than women. The extent to which either gender would take part in voyeurism did depend on how likely they were to be caught, and in this study the highest likelihood that was presented to the participants as a possibility was 25%, which might explain the higher rates compared to the population estimates. Perhaps in real voyeuristic situations people have a much higher expectation of being caught or have some understanding of the potential consequences, whether caught by the people being viewed or by the law. Or perhaps we are more likely to feel a sense of guilt if we are actually doing something as opposed to only imagining doing something (to an extent this has been examined by exploring differences between imagined guilt and recollected guilt—see Mclatchie, Giner-Sorolla, & Derbyshire, 2016). Some support for the idea that there are important concerns regarding comparisons of what people predict they would do and what people actually do is provided by a study by Templeman and Stinnett (1991) who found that in a sample of male college students 42% said that they had engaged in voyeurism. However, that the prevalence is so high is interesting and supports the view of Forsyth (1996) who offered the idea that it might be more useful to think of voyeurism, to some extent, as normal behaviour; given the opportunity to look, most people will look.

A missing element to these estimates is asking people *why* participants would take part in these behaviours. Our expectation might be that the explanation would be almost entirely sexual, that it would provide either immediate or later material to be used for masturbation or for some kind of fantasy. However, such explanations may be dependent on the individual's maturational stage, sexual experience, and their views about their own body or that of their sexual partner, amongst others. A young boy or sexually inexperienced adult who has not seen a naked women may be motivated by curiosity rather than any sexual motivation, as might a young girl or sexually inexperienced woman, and a person with limited sexual experience may be motivated to watch a couple engage in sex to compare their own sexual behaviours with those of others. Is the motivation that lies behind the behaviour important? Perhaps a thought experiment is worth considering. People who frequent art galleries will have seen patrons who will sit for extended periods of time looking at a particular painting. Why do they do that? Perhaps they are an art student who is trying to understand the use of colour, brush techniques, or someone who is emotionally moved by the grandeur and complexity of a particular work. That being the case, we would be unlikely to begrudge them taking up a seat or standing in front of a painting. What if they found the painting sexually stimulating (which might be termed *iconophilia*), either at the time and were surreptitiously pleasuring themselves or were using their memory of the picture for fantasy purposes when they returned to work or home? For a case where art was found to be sexually arousing, see Case 3 in Leiblum and Nathan (2001). The purpose of this experiment is to consider what is it about voyeurism that makes it deviant, is it the looking, is it the invasion of privacy, is it our concern that we have been seen doing something embarrassing, or is it based on our assumptions about what people use that visual information for? This may help us understand the earlier issue regarding the differences in gender. If men and women engage in voyeurism to the same extent, but men are more likely to get caught and then men are more likely to be labelled as being voyeurs, and are more likely condemned for it, is this because we suspect that men are far more likely to have deviant motivations than women or that deviant motivations in men are more deviant, or that the expression of the same deviant motivations, for example masturbation, is considered more sexually deviant or dangerous when performed by men than when performed by women? This would be a useful area to carry out research.

Voyeurism and Other Risks

It is unclear the extent to which voyeurism may be a preparatory phase for other offences, such as sexual assault, or a component of other offences, such as stalking or theft. So, the level of risk implied by voyeurism is unknown, despite studies suggesting that there may be a link (Freund, Scher, Racansky, Campbell, & Heasman, 1986). Hirschfield (1948) reported that voyeurs would frequently watch couples in Paris and then would steal from them, but it is not clear if the voyeurism was simply observation prior to the theft or if the theft was an opportunistic consequence of the voyeurism. Other case studies suggest that voyeurism and sexual offences involving children may be linked but again it is unclear if the two can be separated (see Hammer, 1968). Longo and Groth (1983) found that in their sample of 128 child molesters, 20% were found at interview and from their medico-legal histories to have engaged in voyeurism as children. In their sample of 103 rapists, 24% were found to have been childhood voyeurs. As interesting as these findings are, one must be cautious when thinking about the classification here: do the children meet the definition of voyeur or were they opportunists who happened to be caught watching their neighbours get undressed or having sex, and even if not opportunists, what was the motivation that drove their behaviour?

Abel and colleagues (1987) found that in their sample of 1170 participants who identified as having a paraphilia, 62 identified as voyeurs and of these only 1.5% could be classified as pure voyeurs, that is, with no other paraphilias. For this group, the average number of paraphilias was approximately five, which included behaviours such as rape (23 of the voyeurs), exhibitionism ($n=39$), and female non-incestuous paedophilia ($n = 32$). Does this tell us anything about the development of voyeurism or what it might lead to? There could be a relationship, but is it causal or a developmental stage that is passed through on the way to the eventual form of offending, based on some underlying sexual issue, such as preoccupation or lack of control? This idea is known as the Courtship Disorder Hypothesis (Freund, 1990), which suggests that the patterns of escalation within normal dating relationships, such as finding a potential partner, interacting with that partner prior to physical contact, establishing physical contact, and sexual intercourse, are mirrored in the behaviour of sexual offenders; voyeurism, exhibitionism, frotteurism, and rape (McNally & Fremouw, 2014). We don't know if voyeurism is a stage just as we do not know if sexual assault is a stage that will eventually lead to rape, although research is beginning to examine the pathways of different kinds of offenders, whether they de-escalate, remain stable, or escalate (Wynn & Duff, 2016). However, it is an important area to explore as earlier authors have identified escalation in voyeurs (de River, 1956;

Yalom, 1960), and Yalom (1960) suggests that there are behaviours that may be indicative of voyeurs who will escalate, namely the entering of a building to view a victim (it is not clear if this is the same building that the victim is in or that it is the level of risk and planning implied by entering any building) and drawing the attention of their victims to themselves whilst watching. Also, psychoanalytic theorists have suggested that sadism may be a factor in voyeurism as it can be degrading for the victims (for example, in the case of *coprophilia*; Rosen, 1967) and that in the case of female voyeurs underlying motivations include rage and sadism (Slovenko, 1965).

Understanding the Victim

The second reason to understand more about voyeurism is because of the impact on victims. Although many victims will not know that they are victims, what Landau and Freeman-Longo (1990) refer to as "ignorance of victimisation" in their multidimensional victim typology, the impact of being a target of voyeurism has been minimally explored. Simon (1997) provides a description of the psychological impact on victims discovering that they have been filmed including humiliation, undermining their sense of safety, and in some cases requiring treatment. Most examples of victim impact are in the media and include reports of panic attacks and feeling that one's privacy has been violated (Columbus Dispatch, 2013; *Los Angeles Times*, 2015).

> "Voyeurism affects women in the same ways all forms of violence, harassment and sexism affect women," Westendorf said. "Women are denied ownership and agency of their own bodies." (*The Toronto Observer*, 14 October 2012)

The little that we do know of impact suggests that it has lasting consequences for victims, and thus, understanding voyeurism in order to reduce recidivism has important implications for social health.

Available data do suggest that some people do know that they are victims of voyeurism and are concerned enough to report it. The National Crime Statistics of 2010 suggest that between April 2016 and March 2017, there were 8973 offences of voyeurism or exhibitionism reported to the police, a 10% increase from the same period 2015 to 2016.

One important contradiction to this view that voyeurism is harmful is that of Doyle (2009) who argues that undetected voyeurism is not wrong. He refers to "perfect voyeurism" where a person is viewed or listened to, and yet this is never discovered and is never shared. In this situation, Doyle still believes that it is not wrong regardless of whether the victim(s) would prefer not to be watched or heard. One can certainly see the appeal of the argument; if you are being watched when you next bathe, but do not know at the time and never find out, what harm has befallen you? You have enjoyed a pleasurable bath and your voyeur perhaps has pleasured himself, so everyone is happy and no one is harmed. My concern with this line of argument is what happens (potentially) if we use it in other areas of offending? If a child is too young to understand or report having been sexually abused and there is no physical or emotional harm done, is this "perfect child abuse" doing no harm and as such is not a bad thing? If an adult is unable to communicate through disability, such as Intellectual Disability, that they have been groomed and consequently take part in sexual activity with a member of their care team, and no physical or emotional harm is done, is this behaviour that is technically not of concern? If X happens and no one knows that X has happened, except the person who did it, should we care and what does it mean if we do care (we still, presumably, don't know that it happened)? This is something of a tangent, but does raise some interesting issues about behaviour, and perhaps is particularly pertinent when thinking of voyeurism, where it is entirely possible that much of it goes on without anyone knowing, save the perpetrator, and he/she doesn't mind because that's what he/she wants. Given the high numbers of self-reporting participants who state that they would be voyeurs if they would not be caught, and the relatively low numbers of reports of voyeurism perhaps we have to accept that there is likely a great deal of perfect voyeurism that is going on, but to what extent does this possibility impact on our lives? Perhaps very little, until you read the preceding paragraph.

Public Views of Voyeurs

As with many areas that are related to unusual or undesired behaviour, the public do have a view of voyeurism; however, there are few research studies that have explored this area (see below). This is an important area because the public, either currently are or in the future may be, victims or perpetrators of voyeurism. If the public view of victims is that they are ignored, that if there is a prosecution they cease to become victims but become witnesses to be harshly treated under cross-examination in court, if the voyeur is convicted they get a short sentence and no intervention so they become more risky, will future victims come forward? If the public view of voyeurism is that it does no harm, one is unlikely to get caught, if caught seldom prosecuted, there is little to prevent people slipping into voyeuristic behaviours. Also, if the public do not understand what voyeurism is, they are unlikely to recognise it in themselves and perhaps attempt to prevent it or to seek intervention before it becomes troublesome. We know from research in stalking and sexual offending that public views are seldom the same as legal or psychological views with regard to what counts as troublesome, risky, or warning behaviours (Challinor, 2015; Duff & Scott, 2013), so there is good reason to suspect the same will be true of voyeurism. Where do these views come from? There are a number of likely candidates, though the extent to which they are interrelated or may lead from one to the other is not known.

One important possibility for where views of voyeurism may come from is our own views of what is reasonable and normal, and this is likely informed by discussions with our peers, exposure to media, and our own view of the world. Studies (e.g. Fox, Nobles, & Akers, 2011) have demonstrated that many of our views regarding stalking are informed by the views of our peers, and these tend to be views that minimise the seriousness of it and the harm it might do. If we believe that our curiosity needs to be satisfied, we need some visual material for our fantasies, that it does no harm (and keep in mind Doyle's [2009] idea of perfect voyeurism), we may be more likely to take advantage of opportunities to watch or to seek out targets. The media also play an important role, both in identifying the negative nature of voyeurism (*The Sun*, 23 November 2017) and portraying it as titillating (*The Sun*, 27 February 2018). There have been YouTube channels that focus on different aspects of voyeurism, including "upskirting" (anonymously taking pictures up women's skirts and dresses—which to date is not illegal in the UK), celebrities caught climbing out of cars and flashing their underwear or lack thereof, and the theft of pictures and videos from private stores that are then published on sites such as *Celebrity Jihad* and *Porn Hub*. Exposure to such material may act to inspire people to do similar, either for their own ends or to gain popularity and notoriety on Internet forums (such as the now defunct *Creepshots*) and sites. In some cases, the forums provide instruction to novices, so clearly there are examples where people are encouraging others, either directly or indirectly, to become active in or more accomplished at voyeurism. The below material are excerpts taken from a post that first appeared in the *Creepshots* forum;

> I use full sized cameras. Better image quality and most people pay you no attention when you have one…If you look like you know what you are doing, most people will ignore you. DSLR. By far my favorite camera for creepshots. Why? Because you DO NOT HIDE IT. You can't really, it's too big…The way my SLR hangs on me leaves it at the perfect "aim at the hiney height". I just need walk near a sexy booty, press the trigger and bam, I have a 5 shot per second burst of insanely high quality shots of said booty…Down side: Shutter noise on my current system. Newer cameras give the option to turn this noise off for truly silent photography. So, in the mean time, sneaky shots need to be taken around places with lots of masking background noise. Streets, festivals, etc. (from https://www.reddit.com/r/toronto/comments/113rvn/a_warning_to_the_women_of_toronto/)

For the vulnerable or the curious, these kinds of instructions may both provide the technical know-how and the sense that other people are doing it too, which has been identified as a technique that people use to transfer responsibility of their own actions onto a larger group of people (Coleman, 1987). There may also be an element of their being a "cachet" to being a successful voyeur, one is being "sneaky" and "clandestine" and in that way bettering other people. And after all, as the above example suggests, it's just a picture of "a sexy booty".

As with many other areas of human behaviour, popular film has depicted various aspects of voyeurism. *The Susan Wilson Story* captures an account of the true story of Susan Wilson who was subjected to video voyeurism (a similar idea is presented in *Alone with Her* and as part of *Sliver*) and a variety of films focus on men spying on women using telescopes and binoculars (*Body Double, Disturbia, Rear Window*); an interesting example of this, which is based on the religious diktat not to commit adultery, is the film *Decalogue 6* where a young man spies on a woman but when the opportunity arises to have sex with her he refuses. She seduces him and he then attempts suicide. *One Hour Photo* presents a man who satisfies his voyeurism through making double-copies of a family's photographs, one set to keep for himself, and *American Beauty* has a variety of voyeuristic elements that bring characters to unfortunate ends. The film *Peeping Tom* is not, as one might expect, so much about voyeurism as we are thinking about it here but rather it is about a man who wants to capture the looks on people's faces when they know they are going to die, when he is killing them. What these films have broadly in common is that voyeurism is presented as obsessional, linked to some kind of mental health issue, and ultimately results in tragedy either for the voyeur or the victim, and often bystanders are caught in the crossfire. From the examples I am aware of voyeurism is presented as an exclusively heterosexual behaviour, where females are victims (although there are films where female voyeurism is not covert, such as *Magic Mike* and where female voyeurism is not the central feature of the film, such as *Elle*, or the British Film *Red Road* where the female voyeur is employed to watch CCTV as a security guard). This final factor is perhaps the most interesting, from the perspective of how the public develop their views; potentially only men are seen as "real" voyeurs and either women don't do it or if they do, then it is something other than voyeurism. It is then hard to separate out other gendered biases, particularly related to sexuality and sexual offending, from one's view of voyeurism, i.e. that men are perpetrators, their motives are sexually deviant, and women are victims. Added to this is the concern of risk (although the extent to which people believe that they have been a victim of voyeurism has not been explored) whereby women will only think that they are at risk from men. Although the statistics bear out that this is most likely, we know that there are female voyeurs.

As a final example of the potential for media bias, there is song. Two examples will be provided, *Watching You* by The Outfield ("Did you save your last dance for me? Watching you, Watching you, Know how much I want it, Just watching you") and The Police's *Every Breath You Take* ("Every breath you take, Every move you make, Every bond you break, Every step you take, I'll be watching you"); in both cases, the watching of someone is romanticised and presented as evidence of longing and love. This is not to suggest that these are not intended as love songs (although they may not be), and that paying attention to what someone does, wanting to dance with them, isn't romantic. However, it is also plausible that in so doing, for some people, the sensitivity to another's behaviour when it is of this kind may be affected so that people are more tolerant than may be ideal and some people may learn behaviours in this way, assuming that they are considered by society to be romantic and harmless. We may be more likely to initially interpret our own and others' behaviour as positive. Of course care has to be taken not to pathologise everything that could be interpreted as promoting unpleasant or harmful behaviour and see every song and every film as warping the minds of the youth or the vulnerable. We could, however, find out if our views of voyeurism are impacted upon by the media and identify ways to prevent it if it is a problem.

Furnham has undertaken a range of studies asking the public what they believe are the most important factors in the development and cure of a range of problematic conditions (e.g. Furnham 1989; Furnham & McDermott, 1994). The motivation for these studies is Furnham's view (1988) that there are similarities between the explicit theories of academia and the implicit theories held by laypeople and as such lay theories may provide some useful insights in understanding phenomena. A secondary consequence of this view is that lay theories may underpin the thoughts and behaviours of those who are labelled as delinquent or alcoholic and may be important in understanding the extent to which an individual may feel their thoughts and actions are within or without their control. Furnham has taken this same approach with paraphilias, and within that has explored public views concerning voyeurism (Furnham & Haraldsen, 1998). In this study, the findings indicated that for voyeurism, as with the other paraphilias under consideration (fetishism, paedophilia, and sexual sadism), the factors identified as most important for its development were fearing the opposite sex, having been a victim of child abuse, experiencing strict parenting, and possessing repressed sexual feelings. The results also indicated that the factors which differentiate voyeurism from the other three paraphilias are early relationships (abuse and early sexual experiences), repressed emotions (including lack of empathy in childhood), and biology (physiological factors). The fact that the general public have a view and that the factors they identify could be classified as external and societal as opposed to internal and biological for the development of voyeurism is interesting and worthy of a degree of speculation. It might suggest that we generally believe that voyeurs are made and not born (which is interesting given that there is evidence that much of our visual preference is present very early on (Morton & Johnson, 1991; Pascalis, de Schonen, Morton, Deruelle, & Fabre-Grenet, 1995). For the sample in the study that may have identified as voyeurs, it allows them to blame others and for those who don't want to identify their behaviour as voyeuristic they can blame external factors that they know they have not experienced. This is a cynical view of the findings but presumably there is an explanation for any of these particular explanatory descriptions that are offered by laypeople, just as there are when we examine laypersons' theories of physics (McCloskey & Kohl, 1983). So care needs to be taken when we take the views of others entirely at face value, without considering there may be some complex thinking that lies behind the expression of our own and others' views.

As mentioned earlier, the public, we, are voyeurs and the public, we, are victims of voyeurism, and understanding this lay-stance on voyeurism may be useful for thinking about prevalence, risk, and, from the perspective of the voyeurs, treatability; if they think nothing can be done, they might not seek help or engage with it if it is Court-mandated (see Walton and Duff [2017] for the views of sex offenders who struggle to believe that they can change). Unless otherwise demonstrated, a good starting point for understanding someone and their behaviour is that they are a person, like us.

So having considered the views of the public, how has psychology tried to understand voyeurism to date?

References

Abel, G. G., Becker, J. V., Mittelman, M., Cunningham-Rather, J., Rouleau, J. L., & Murphy, W. D. (1987). Self-reported sex crimes of nonincarcerated paraphiliacs. *Journal of Interpersonal Violence, 2*(1), 3–25.

Abouesh, A., & Clayton, A. (1999). Compulsive voyeurism and exhibitionism: A clinical response to paroxetine. *Archives of Sexual Behavior, 28*(1), 23–30.

Ahlers, C. J., Schaefer, G. A., Mundt, I. A., Roll, S., Englert, H., Willich, S. N., et al. (2011). How unusual are the contents of the paraphilias? Paraphilia-associated sexual arousal patterns in a community-based sample of men. *Journal of Sexual Medicine, 8,* 1362–1370.

Allen, C. (1969). *A textbook of psychosexual disorders* (2nd ed.). London: Oxford University Press.

American Psychiatric Association. (2000). *Diagnostic and statistical manual of mental disorders* (4th ed., text revision). Washington, DC: Author.

Challinor, L. (2015). The perceptions of sex offenders: A comparison of professionals and paraprofessionals in a forensic environment and the general public. *Forensic Update, 117,* 32–36.

Coleman, J. T. (1987). Toward an integrated theory of white-collar crime. *American Journal of Sociology, 93*(2), 406–439.

Columbus Dispatch. (2013). Retrieved November 10, 2016, from http://www.dispatch.com/content/stories/public/2013/08/15/dibble-sentenced.html.

Dawson, S. J., Bannerman, B. A., & Lalumière, M. (2016). Paraphilic interests: An examination of sex differences in a nonclinical sample. *Sex Abuse: A Journal of Treatment and Research, 28*(1), 20–45.

de Oliveira, W. M., Jr., & Abdo, C. H. N. (2010). Unconventional sexual behaviors and their associations with physical, mental and sexual health parameters: A study in 18 large Brazilian cities. *Revista Brasileira de Psiquiatria, 32*(3), 264–274.

de River, J. P. (1956). *The sexual criminal.* Springfield, IL: Charles C. Thomas.

Doyle, T. (2009). Privacy and perfect voyeurism. *Ethics and Information Technology, 11*, 181–189.

Duff, S. C., & Scott, A. J. (2013). Understanding perceptions of stalking: The impact of additional contextual information regarding the breakdown of relationships. *Journal of Criminal Psychology, 3*(2), 136–144.

Forsyth, C. J. (1996). The structuring of vicarious sex. *Deviant Behavior, 17*(3), 279–295.

Fox, K. A., Nobles, M. R., & Akers, R. L. (2011). Is stalking a learned phenomenon? An empirical test of social learning theory. *Journal of Criminal Justice, 39*(1), 39–47.

Freund, K. (1990). Courtship disorder. In W. L. Marshall, D. R. Laws, & H. E. Barbaree (Eds.), *Handbook of sexual assault: Issues, theories and treatment of the offender* (pp. 195–207). New York: Plenum Press.

Freund, K., Scher, H., Racansky, I. G., Campbell, K., & Heasman, G. (1986). Males disposed to commit rape. *Archives of Sexual Behavior, 15*(1), 23–35.

Furnham, A. (1988). *Lay theories.* Oxford: Pergamon.

Furnham, A. (1989). Overcoming 'psychosomatic' illness: Lay attributions of cure for five possible psychosomattc illnesses. *Social Science and Medicine, 29*, 61–67.

Furnham, A., & Haraldsen, E. (1998). Lay theories of etiology and "cure" for four types of paraphilia: Fetishism; Pedophilia; sexual sadism and voyeurism. *Journal of Clinical Psychology, 54*(5), 689–700.

Furnham, A., & McDermott, M. R. (1994). Lay beliefs about the efficacy of self-reliance, seeking help, and external control as strategies for overcoming obesity, drug addiction, marital problems, stuttering, and insomnia. *Psychology and Health, 9*, 397–406.

Gebhard, P. H., Gagnon, J. H., Pomeroy, W. B., & Christenson, C. V. (1965). *Sex offenders.* New York: Harper & Row.

Hammer, E. F. (1968). Symptoms of sexual deviation: Dynamics and etiology. *Psychoanalytic Review, 55*, 5–27.

Hirschfield, M. (1948). *Sexual anomalies and perversions.* London: Francis Alder.

Hocken, K., & Thorne, K. (2012). Voyeurism, exhibitionism and other non-contact sexual offences. In B. Winder & P. Banyard (Eds.), *A psychologist's casebook of crime: From arson to voyeurism.* Houndsmills, UK: Palgrave Macmillan.

Hopkins, T. A., Green, B. A., Carnes, P. J., & Campling, S. (2016). Varieties of intrusion: Exhibitionism and voyeurism. *Sexual Addiction & Compulsivity, 23*(1), 4–33.

Joyal, C. C., & Carpentier, J. (2016). The prevalence of paraphilic interests and behaviors in the general population: A provincial survey. *The Journal of Sex Research, 54*(2), 161–171.

Kaplan, M., & Krueger, R. (1997). Voyeurism: Psychopathology and theory. In D. R. Laws & W. O'Donohue (Eds.), *Sexual deviance: Theory, assessment, and treatment* (pp. 297–310). New York, NY: Guilford Press.

Landau, S. F., & Freeman-Longo, R. E. (1990). Classifying victims: A proposed multidimensional victimological typology. *International Review of Victimology, 1,* 267–286.

Långström, N., & Seto, M. C. (2006). Exhibitionistic and voyeuristic behaviour in a Swedish national population sample. *Archives of Sexual Behavior, 35,* 427–435.

Leiblum, S. R., & Nathan, S. G. (2001). Persistent sexual arousal syndrome: A newly discovered pattern of female sexuality. *Journal of Sex & Marital Therapy, 27*(4), 365–380.

Longo, R. E., & Groth, A. N. (1983). Juvenile sexual offences in the histories of adult rapists and child molesters. *International Journal of Offender Therapy and Comparative Criminology, 27,* 150–155.

Los Angeles Times. (2015). Retrieved November 10, 2017, from http://www.latimes.com/local/crime/la-me-hollywood-video-voyeur-20150802-story.html.

Makanjuola, A. B., Adegunloye, O. A., & Adelekan, M. L. (2008). Disorders of sexual preference among secondary school teachers in Ilorin, Nigeria. *Nigerian Journal of Psychiatry, 6*(1), 26–30.

Maletzky, B. M., & McGovern, K. B. (1991). *Treating the sexual offender.* Newbury Park: Sage.

Mann, R. E., Ainsworth, F., Al-Attar, Z., & Davies, M. (2008). Voyeurism: Assessment and treatment. In D. R. Laws & W. T. O'Donohue (Eds.), *Sexual Deviance* (2nd ed., pp. 320–335). New York: Guilford Press.

Marsh, P. J., Odlaug, B. L., Thomarios, N., Davis, A. A., Buchanan, S. N., Meyer, C. S., & Grant, J. E. (2010). Paraphilias in adult psychiatric inpatients. *Annals of Clinical Psychiatry, 22*(2), 129–134.

McCloskey, M., & Kohl, D. (1983). Naïve physics: The curvilinear impetus principle and its role in interactions with moving objects. *Journal of Experimental Psychology: Learning, Memory, & Cognition, 9*(1), 146–156.

Mclatchie, N., Giner-Sorolla, R., & Derbyshire, S. W. G. (2016). 'Imagined guilt' vs 'recollect guilt': Implications for fMRI. *Social and Affective Neuroscience, 11*(5), 703–711.

McNally, M. R., & Fremouw. W. J. (2014). Examining risk of escalation: A critical review of the exhibitionistic behavior literature. *Aggression and Violent Behavior, 19*(5), 474–485.

Morton, J., & Johnson, M. H. (1991). CONSPEC and CONLERN: A two process theory of infant face recognition. *Psychology Review, 2,* 164–181.

Pascalis, O., de Schonen, S., Morton, J., Deruelle, C., & Fabre-Grenet, M. (1995). Mother's face recognition by neonates: A replication and an extension. *Infant Behavior Development, 18,* 79–95.

Rosen, I. (1967). *Pathology and treatment of sexual deviations.* Oxford: Oxford University Press.

Rye, B. J., & Meaney, G. J. (2007). Voyeurism. *International Journal of Sexual Health, 19*(1), 47–56.

Simon, R. I. (1997). Video voyeurs and the covert videotaping of unsuspecting victims: Psychological and legal consequences. *Journal of Forensic Science, 42*(5), 884–889.

Slovenko, R. (1965). *Sexual behavior and the law.* Springfield, IL: Charles C. Thomas.

Smith, R. S. (1976). Voyeurism: A literature review. *Archives of Sexual Behavior, 5*(6), 585–608.

Templeman, T. L., & Stinnett, R. D. (1991). Patterns of sexual arousal and history in a "normal" sample of young men. *Archives of Sexual Behavior, 20,* 137–150.

The Sun. (2017, November 23). Retrieved February 28, 2018, from https://www.thesun.co.uk/news/4970233/man-hid-secret-camera-starbucks-toilet-south-london/.

The Toronto Observer. (2012, October 14). Retrieved February 28, 2018, from https://torontoobserver.ca/2012/10/14/voyeur-websites-under-scrutiny-by-police-and-public/.

Walton, J. S., & Duff, S. (2017). "I'm not homosexual or heterosexual, I'm paedosexual": Exploring sexual preference for children using interpretive phenomenology. *Journal of Forensic Practice, 19*(2), 151–161.

Wynn, C., & Duff, S. (2016). *Offence Patterns in Repeat Sexual Offenders: An examination of escalation, de-escalation, and stability across sexual offence categories.* Division of Forensic Psychology Annual Conference, Manchester Metropolitan University, England, June 2016.

Yalom, I. D. (1960). Aggression and forbiddenness in voyeurism. *Archives of General Psychiatry, 3*(3), 305–319.

CHAPTER 4

Explanations of Voyeurism

Abstract This chapter summarises a variety of explanations for the development and maintenance of voyeurism including psychoanalytic theories, learning theories, and neuropsychological theories.

Keywords Psychoanalysis · Neuropsychology · "Innate releasing mechanism" (IRM) · "Up-skirting"

A comprehensive theory of voyeurism does not exist, rather ideas have been offered as potential explanations and often these have not been fully examined. More often than not it is because of the ethical issues of conducting empirical studies where we may be exposing people to stimuli that might lead them to behave in ways that could be distressing for them, distressing for others, and result in criminal offending. It is also important to consider that the majority of hypotheses offered have been more generally considered for behaviour of a general fetishistic kind rather than specifically for voyeurism. So, when thinking about these hypotheses it would be best to consider that they may explain why sexualised looking becomes important because of the meaning of what is looked at, to that individual, rather than that the behaviour of "looking" per se becomes more prevalent or important.

For each of the approaches considered below, a degree of critique will be offered. This should not be interpreted as trying to intentionally force a particular theoretical viewpoint on the reader, but rather to

S. Duff, *Voyeurism*, https://doi.org/10.1007/978-3-319-97160-5_4

critically engage with the thinking of these approaches. As we are not at a point where there is a good explanatory model for voyeurism, it is too early to think that each of these approaches may not offer something to our understanding and possibly provide interesting avenues for further exploration.

Psychoanalytic Explanations

Numerous psychoanalytic explanations have been offered developing from Freud's original ideas in 1938. His view was that child sexuality is made up of a number of impulses that result in identifying others as the focus of sexual behaviour, and one of these impulses is to look. With maturation, the various impulses become integrated into adult sexuality. However, it is possible that an impulse could become independent and thus the individual may have their typical sexual drive along with a drive to satisfy this second impulse, or this secondary impulse may, over time, become more important. Thus, either an individual may have a healthy sexual life and also be a voyeur, or they may be primarily a voyeur and have a less satisfactory sexual life, or no interest in other forms of sexual expression.

Other examples of psychoanalytic explanations for fetishism and voyeurism include the psychoanalytic approach of Sperling (1963) who suggested that fetishism in childhood was an attempt to gain gratifications that could not be obtained from the child's mother. From Freud's view, that fetishism is the "after-effect of some sexual impression, received as a rule in early childhood" (Freud, 1977, pp. 351–352); the implication is that the gratification is of a sexual nature. Lorand and Schneer (1967) concluded that the adult's sexual aims during voyeurism are the aims of a child. This does rely on accepting the idea that children are "sexual" and seek sexual gratification and that early sexual impressions can have a lasting effect. What these sexual impressions might be and at what age they can have an effect are not clear.

Psychoanalytic explanations have linked voyeurism to castration anxiety (Fenichel, 1945). Friedman (1959) was of the opinion that all voyeurism could be interpreted as the individual seeking reassurance against castration anxiety. This would imply that only males will demonstrate voyeurism (this is not entirely true as the idea is that females experience castration anxiety when they realise that they don't have a penis and thus are inclined to search for penises in the world as that would help females manage their assumed feelings of inferiority). As an example, in the case of *coprophilia* the explanation provided, relating to castration anxiety, is that the voyeur is attempting to satisfy their need to see that something resembling a penis does come from a woman's body (where the faeces are assumed to be equivalent in this thinking to a penis, Fenichel, 1945). Other authors have suggested that similar satisfaction could be gained by seeing a woman's breasts because the breast can also symbolise the penis, on the basis that both are "fluid giving organs" (Smith, 1976, p. 588). Later psychoanalytic theories have specifically suggested that voyeurism is an expression of a need to resolve inner conflicts, co-occurring with a lack of control over sexual behaviour (Rye & Meaney, 2007).

These are understandably difficult to test as we cannot easily rely on the recollections of adults as to what gratification they sought as children or what would count as a "sexual impression". Additionally, we need to consider the evidence for phenomena such as castration anxiety (see Schwartz, 1956, for one example). A useful source for examining the testing of Freudian ideas in general, along with critiques, can be found in Eysenck and Wilson's (2013) book. So how useful is this approach? Perhaps most useful is that it highlights the idea that early influences may play an important role in our sexual behaviour and that it is plausible that we are more vulnerable to these influences at particular developmental stages.

Instinctual Explanations

As mentioned earlier, sexual behaviour is an expression of both our genetics and our experiences. At the most basic level, one cannot be a cisgender straight, or bisexual, or lesbian "woman" unless one is a female, and being female, typically, includes a variety of genetic pre-determinants that impact on behaviour, even if by morphology alone. It is also reasonable to assume that our adult sexual repertoire is at least partly informed by a combination of influences from caregivers and friends, things our partners have asked us to do or let us do, and through educational, entertainment, and pornographic media. When these experiences occur during a particular life stage and impact on us, it is known as "imprinting". Typically we think of imprinting taking place in youth, and there is evidence of different examples of imprinting amongst young animals, notably the work of Lorenz (see Vicedo, 2009) who had birds follow him on the ground, which was extended by D'Arrigo (2006) by imprinting birds to fly alongside him. The idea is that animals have instincts for particular kinds of behaviours and in the normal course of events, these instincts will be expressed "normally"; thus, birds will follow birds, not men, and people will have sex with people, not with animals or sofas. In relation to voyeurism, it has been suggested that sexual behaviour is also instinctive, and that the normal instinctive expression of sexuality is that of intercourse between people of opposite sexes and of similar ages (so quite a restricted view of human sexuality; see Pinkava, 1971). Instinctive sexuality occurs when the necessary "innate releasing mechanism" (IRM) is activated by a particular stimulus, and this IRM also includes a description of what are considered suitable targets for sexualised behaviour. Where this mechanism can go wrong is if the specification of the "targets" becomes either too broad, so might include, for example, animals, or becomes too specific, and thus might be exclusive to particular items of clothing, or if the range of target behaviours that are included in that description of the instinctual response become too broad or too narrow. Smith (1976) suggests that voyeurism can occur when the instinctual behaviour includes, or may consist solely of, looking.

Imprinting has been observed in relation to sexual behaviour, whereby male goats brought up by sheep and vice versa showed a mating preference for the other species rather than their own (Kendrick, Hinton, Atkins, Haupt, & Skinner, 1998). This was found to remain for 3 years, even though the animals were later living with their own species. A study has sought to examine the possible impact of imprinting on human sexuality that manages to avoid the ethical problem of performing potentially damaging experiments on young children. Enquist and colleagues (2011) examined sexual imprinting in humans, specifically in men and women who find pregnant and/or lactating women sexually attractive. They recruited this sample from a variety of online forums, and the sample self-identified as having this interest. The researchers investigated if there was a relationship between this self-identified sexual interest and having been exposed to a pregnant and/or lactating mother during early childhood, by the existence of younger siblings; the idea being that such exposure might influence adult sexual interests. The researchers did find such a relationship in both males and females, although there were more males who self-identified with this interest. This is an interesting finding as it suggests that early exposure, not necessarily to traumatic experiences and not necessarily sexual experiences (this is my personal, adult view. Perhaps for a young child seeing one's mother pregnant and/or breast feeding may be interpreted as traumatic or somehow sexual), may impact on sexual development, although the mechanism of this is not identified. It is important to note that the relationship is an association, not causal, as it is plausible that particular children would have eventually been sexually attracted to lactating/pregnant women without any exposure. Presumably this could be tested. For the female participants, it raises an intriguing question. The researchers did ask participants their sexual preference but this is not provided in the analysis, but is it possible that this exposure not only led females to become sexually attracted to lactation or pregnancy, but also to women? If imprinting occurs and can influence sexual attraction in humans, then there are a variety of other studies that could be carried out. For example, could one investigate the impact of children, male and female, having seen their parent(s) naked, having sex, using the toilet, and determine if this has an effect on later expressions of sexuality? This would require that the parents are able to provide the evidence of having been seen by their child as few of us can remember with any accuracy our very early experiences.

Most importantly, in Enquist's study early exposure was not associated with a sexual preference in all of the children, male or female, so there must be some vulnerability or other events that were present during the period of exposure for some of those children, which would lead to this association. Frequently, theories suggest that those "other events" are of a sexual nature, such as the child may be touching their genitals at the same time and thus the experiences that they are exposed to become linked to feelings of pleasure (e.g. Snaith, 1983). Ultimately though, it appears that a specific form of early exposure can lead to a specific form of sexual interest, so it is plausible there could be some kind of exposure that could have a relationship with voyeurism.

Imprinting ideas are interesting as they suggest that early experience of particular kinds may be important for biasing our behaviour in particular ways. From the evidence, it seems that there may be other important concomitant factors that also need to exist, or some kind of vulnerability, and it is these that will be a challenge to identify. However, they reinforce the idea that early experiences are important, in some people, for determining some of the expressions of sexuality.

Neuropsychological Explanations

A number of neuropsychological theories have suggested reductions in control of sexual behaviour as an explanation for voyeurism, specifically that brain damage may result in individuals finding it harder to repress sexual motivations and thus voyeurism may occur (Briken, Habermann, Berner, & Hill, 2005). This implies that voyeurism, amongst other paraphilias, is typically repressed rather than acquired, which does fit with some theories explaining sexual offending (and some psychoanalytic theories). For example, regarding their integrated theory of sexual offending Marshall and Barbaree (1990) write, "…biological inheritance confers upon males a ready capacity to sexually aggress which must be overcome by appropriate training to instill social inhibitions toward such behaviour" (pp. 270–271). This suggests that the problem that the brain damage inflicts is either upon the learning of whatever acts to instil social inhibitions or supports the expression of them. This is important to examine if we are to develop interventions that can work with such a damaged system. However, it is also possible that some children may not develop in an environment where the appropriate repressing material is available and either they do not learn it or they only learn it as adults. We might expect that repression, through training or social pressure, could occur at an early age but we might also expect that the greatest incidents of voyeurism would occur in childhood. They might, but we may not identify this behaviour as troublesome in children or may label it as youthful curiosity. However, circumstances may result in otherwise repressed voyeurism becoming apparent in adults (for example, stressful life events, drug use, trauma) or it may be that only in adults who have not learned the appropriate social rules, or can't express them, does the behaviour become labelled and come to the attention of the authorities or other professionals. As such, it may be difficult to gather evidence to support this particular idea. Evidence of late onset voyeurism (Abel, Obsorn, & Twigg, 1993) in non-brain damaged individuals challenges the idea of voyeurism (assuming that it is truly late onset and with no identifiable triggers) as a consequence of loss of control as does the existence of individuals where voyeurism is the only known example of sexually inappropriate behaviour (unless we are happy with the notion that this kind of loss of control can be very specific).

Learning Theories

As suggested earlier, it is reasonable to think that much of our behaviour, including our sexual behaviour, is learned through observation and direct teaching. This can be both positive, such as in the use of condoms (Caron, Godin, Otis, & Lambert, 2004), and negative, as inter-partner violence (IPV) has been suggested as being at least partly passed through the generations by direct observation (Smith, Ireland, Park, Elwyn, & Thornberry, 2011). A variety of different learning possibilities for voyeurism have been put forward.

One-trial learning suggests that voyeurism (and thus other behaviours considered to be deviant) can be learned through either a single positive experience or through some form of traumatic experience, which may be accidental. However, there is little evidence for one-trial learning linked to unusual sexual behaviour, rather there may be a single event and then that is later used in fantasy (McGuire, Carlisle, & Young, 1964) and reinforced through masturbation. An example of one-trial learning is that offered by Weinberg, Williams, and Calhan (1995) who interviewed homosexual men who self-identified as having a foot fetish. One described the precipitous event thus, "I was home alone and saw my uncle's new penny loafers. I went over and started smelling the fresh new leather scent and kissing and licking them. It turned me on so much that I actually ejaculated my first load into my pants and have been turned on ever since" (p. 23). More frequently learning theories consider classical and instrumental conditioning and there is evidence for both being able to influence sexual behaviour (Abel and Blanchard, 1974; Laws and Marshall, 1990). For example, by pairing erotic pictures with women's boots Rachman and Hodgson (1968) showed that men could learn to develop erections to the women's boots and would eventually respond to the women's boots alone. Similar research paired erotic stimuli with coloured circles and eventually the circles alone were able to elicit erections (McConaghy, 1970). As a final example, men receiving financial reward for becoming aroused to erotic materials could then become aroused in the absence of the erotic stimuli (Rosen, Shapiro, & Schwartz, 1975). That there are learning mechanisms for the development of fetishes and for the occurrence of erections (outside of routine sexual contexts) suggests that other forms of sexual behaviour could similarly develop through this kind of learning process.

Learning theories do have appeal, but it is worth considering how this might happen in the case of the voyeur. If the stimuli are something that is routinely in the environment, such as access to pictures and films of people (having sex, naked, using the toilet, undressing, being seen through windows, portrayed as not knowing they are being seen) and there is a sexual response to those stimuli, then we would either have to accept that voyeurism is far more prevalent than we think or that there are some people who are particularly sensitive to visual stimuli, or perhaps there is a developmental phase during which exposure to visual material can exert an effect with the consequence that voyeurism becomes a concerning behaviour. However, it may also be that it is the pairing of the stimuli, coincidentally, with sexual arousal, which starts the learning process; a male experiences a spontaneous erection at the same time as he sees a woman through a window and the erection is incorrectly paired with the visual scene such that the visual scene is understood by that male as causing the erection. When that male is next in need of some form of fantasy stimulus, he may recall that he found that scene arousing and use it for masturbation, and thus, the coincidental pairing is reinforced. It is not unreasonable to suggest that this person would then seek out other examples of material for later fantasy, particularly if other forms of sexual stimuli have been unsatisfactory or he considers them risky to his self-esteem. In this case for voyeurism to become a part of someone's sexual repertoire not only would there have had to be the initial, coincidental pairing, but also that scene would have to be selected (and possibly routinely and in preference to other fantasies) for later successful sexual stimulation. As to why someone might choose to access fantasy material that was of an unusual nature, McGuire et al. (1964) reported that more than half of their sample of 45 patients (3 voyeurs), whom they described as sexual deviants, reported "that a normal sex life was not possible for them" (p. 186) and that this belief predated the onset of the deviance. In one case they report as follows:

Case 6

This 28-year-old patient, married at the age of 24, had had normal sexual interests. However, his wife proved to be totally frigid so that the marriage was never consummated. In the early months of his marriage, while sexually frustrated, he observed that a young lady in the opposite flat was in the habit of stripping in a lighted room with the curtains open. (The patient's wife confirmed this story.) The patient found this very stimulating

> sexually. The marriage had not been consummated when the couple moved house. In his new environment the patient sought opportunities of seeing women undressing and developed the habit of masturbating on these occasions. (McGuire et al., 1964, p. 189)

The implication is that the man realised that he would never have sexual intercourse and thus had no sexual outlet, nor could he fantasise about intercourse, but he had found another way to have a sexual life.

These ideas are testable, in similar ways that were used to show that people could learn to sexually respond to inanimate objects (Rachman & Hodgson, 1968), but it might not be considered ethical to do so. The clinical advantage of learning theories is that they suggest that voyeurism could also be unlearned, and indeed, a variety of techniques have been tried to help people to unlearn troubling sexual behaviour (see below) although the extent to which they have been successful is not entirely clear.

Another form of learning that has been suggested as potentially linked to voyeurism is social learning. The idea is that we see what other people do, what they value, what they get away with, and we may start to imitate that behaviour (e.g. Bandura, 1965), particularly if we then discover it is beneficial to ourselves. Social learning has been considered useful in understanding examples of stalking behaviours (Fox, Nobles, & Akers, 2011), IPV (Gelles, 1983), and how children learn stereotypical sex role behaviours (Perry & Bussey, 1979), and it may provide a useful explanation for voyeurism. Our own experience tells us that others value viewing people and behaviour, as our friends suggest we look at particular people on the street, or up at a window; there is the cliché, "you can look but you can't touch", which is often part of the negotiated behaviour between couples jokingly reminding one's partner that looking at another man or woman is as far as they are allowed to go. It also implies that looking has "enough" value and that it is sanctioned. As earlier described, the media are full of long-distance photographs of topless celebrities, people getting out of cars, and "up-skirting" and "down-blousing" images. Society and our peers (and us) are communicating that it is OK to look, that if you look you may see things that people might not want you to see, that you may see things that you would otherwise not be able to see. Perhaps most important is that looking does, mostly, provide risk-free access to stimuli that typically involve a degree of risk. If you want to see a particular person naked, normally that would require the risk of meeting them, dating them, and persuading them to get naked. If you are risk averse in general, or particularly to those kinds of social and personal risks, it might be more simple, and just as satisfying, to try to see people naked without that kind of risk. It may allow a particular person that you wish to see naked, or a particular type of person. This would be interesting to examine, if voyeurs are specific in what they wish to see, either the characteristics of the person or the characteristics of the behaviour. Also, looking can be done secretly or remotely, and images can be recorded. For social learning to take place, there need not be immediate rewards (Bandura, 1977), but there can certainly be rewards such as feelings of power, dominance, accomplishment, along with sexual rewards that can occur at a later time.

Other Explanations

Rather than a lack of control of behaviour, Smith (1976) has suggested that voyeurs may find sexual intercourse unsatisfactory or simply have a preference for voyeurism. This is different from a learned response suggesting as it does some kind of predisposition towards voyeurism or away from other forms of sexual activity that are considered normal. The fact that the voyeuristic act is often coupled at the time or later with masturbation would provide suitable positive reinforcement for the behaviour to be repeated. Are there people who do not consider sexual intercourse the most satisfying form of sexual behaviour? This is quite a complex question because we know that a variety of factors play a role in changing people's sexual behaviour, for example age and relationship status (cohabiting couples appear to have more "sex" than married couples or non-cohabiting couples), but this research tends to only look at the frequency of intercourse as a measure of sexual satisfaction. The research that I am aware of does not seem to consider whether a reduction in one kind of available sexual behaviour (for example, intercourse) is paralleled by an increase in another (for example, voyeurism or use of pornography) nor do there seem to be surveys of preference. Indeed, there seems to be an assumption that research concerned with sex is only really concerned with sexual intercourse. As an example, Nicolosi and colleagues (2004) carried out a large study to investigate sexual behaviour and sexual dysfunction in people aged over 40 years. They gathered responses from 27,516 people from countries such as Brazil, Israel, Japan, the USA, and European countries. It is apparent from their results that they only considered, or at best only report, findings related to sexual intercourse, and as such we really cannot be sure what people mean when providing quality of life answers in relation to sexual dysfunction. A man with premature ejaculation may not find intercourse satisfactory but may have found a way to still have a satisfactory sexual quality of life through some other means. As the case cited from McGuire et al. (1964) suggests, if one method of sexual expression is unavailable then another may be found; this does not necessarily mean that he did not find sexual intercourse pleasurable and preferable. This idea, of finding new ways to achieve the same sexual goals, has been referred to as "turn-on patterns" (basically, the things that we find arousing), and it has been suggested that we can learn new sexual turn-on patterns (see Pirelli, Esben, Almås, & Weingarten, 2015).

However, other theories argue that voyeurism may not be linked to any form of underlying pathology. Evolutionary theories suggest that males looking at females is an element of mate selection (Rhodes et al., 2005), which might more easily explain voyeurism if it was not often paired with sexual activity displaced from the target rather than attempting to have sex once the target has been seen and found to be a suitable mate. One explanation for this is that voyeurs find translating the identification of a "potential mate" into an "actual mate" difficult, which may be due to poor social skills or fears of intimacy (Freund and Seto, 1998—what Freund [1988] termed courtship disorder). A second non-pathology approach is that voyeurism is socially managed in that it is a basic drive for us to be interested in people, particularly when they are engaged in typically private activities, but the extent to which this interest is expressed is dependent on social support and learning from others, the extent to which it is likely to be sanctioned by the authorities if one is caught, and how concerned one is about being caught (Kutchinsky, 1976; Rye & Meaney, 2007). Finally, there may be no underlying sexual pathology but issues with social anxiety, which is linked to a variety of sexual offences (Hoyer, Kunst, & Schmidt, 2001), or poor self-esteem (Maletzky, 1991). This view of the development and maintenance of voyeurism being situated within social processes fits with the views of Becker and Kaplan (1988) that individual factors, social factors, and the environment are possible precursors. In a similar, more broad approach, Lavin (2008) suggests that it might be useful to recruit Money's (1986) idea of "lovemaps" although it is not clear if this provides greater insight than considering that sexual behaviour and sexual partners may be represented in schemata that guide sexual preferences and sexual activity. Indeed, a typical cognitive approach to understanding voyeurism is notable by its absence.

The various approaches to increase our understanding of voyeurism have provided some valuable clues and directions for further work. The case study presented here adds further value by focussing on a particular case of voyeurism in an adult male where the process of assessment and intervention identifies a number of important elements in the development and maintenance of voyeurism. The case is particularly interesting as it involves two distinct elements of offending behaviour, "up-skirting" and voyeurism in female toilets.

References

Abel, G. G., & Blanchard, E. B. (1974). The role of fantasy in the treatment of sexual deviation. *Archives of General Psychiatry, 30*, 467–475.

Abel, G. G., Obsorn, C., & Twigg, D. (1993). Sexual assault through the life span: Adult offenders with juvenile histories. In H. E. Barbaree, W. Marshall, & S. M. Hudson (Eds.), *The juvenile sex offender* (pp. 104–117). New York: Guilford Press.

Bandura, A. (1965). Behavior modification through modeling procedures. In L. Krasner, & L. P. Ullman (Eds.), *Research in Behavior Modification*. NY: Holt, Rinehart and Winston.

Bandura, A. (1977). *Social learning theory*. NY: Prentice-Hall.

Becker, J. V., & Kaplan, M. S. (1988). The assessment of adolescent sexual offenders. In R. J. Prinz (Ed.), *Advances in behavioural assessment of children and families* (pp. 97–118). Conn: JAI Press Inc.

Briken, P., Habermann, N., Berner, W., & Hill, A. (2005). The influence of brain abnormalities on psychosocial development, criminal history and paraphilias in sexual murderers. *Journal of Forensic Science, 50*, 1204–1208.

Caron, F., Godin, G., Otis, J., & Lambert, L. D. (2004). Evaluation of a theoretically based AIDS/STD peer education program on postponing sexual intercourse and on condom use among adolescents attending high school. *Health Education Research, 19*(2), 185–197.

D'Arrigo, A. (2006). *L'Homme Oiseau*. Paris: Arthaud.

Enquist, M., Aronsson, H., Ghirlanda, S., Jansson, L., & Jannini, E. A. (2011). Exposure to mother's pregnancy and lactation in infancy is associated with sexual attraction to pregnancy and lactation in adulthood. *Journal of Sexual Medicine, 8*, 140–147.

Eysenck, H. J., & Wilson, G. D. (2013). *The experimental study of Freudian theory*. London: Routledge.

Fenichel, O. (1945). *The psychoanalytic theory of neurosis.* New York: Norton.

Fox, K. A., Nobles, M. R., & Akers, R. L. (2011). Is stalking a learned phenomenon? An empirical test of social learning theory. *Journal of Criminal Justice, 39*(1), 39–47.

Freud, S. (1977). *On sexuality: Three essays on the theory of sexuality and other works.* Harmondsworth: Penguin.

Freund, K. (1988). Courtship disorders: Is this hypothesis valid? *Annals of the New York Academy of Sciences, 528*, 172–182.

Freund, K., & Seto, M. C. (1998). Preferential rape in the theory of courtship disorder. *Archives of Sexual Behavior, 27*, 433–443.

Friedman, P. (1959). Sexual deviations. In S. Arieti (Ed.), *American handbook of psychiatry* (pp. 589–603). New York: Basic Books.

Gelles, R. J. (1983). An exchange/social control theory. In D. Finkelhor, R. J. Gelles, G. Hotaling, & M. A. Straus (Eds.), *The dark side of families* (pp. 182–192). Beverly Hills, CA: Sage.

Hoyer, J., Kunst, H., & Schmidt, A. (2001). Social phobia as a comorbid condition in sex offenders with paraphilia or impulse control disorder. *The Journal of Nervous and Mental Disease, 189*(7), 463–470.

Kendrick, K. M., Hinton, M. R., Atkins, K., Haupt, M. A., & Skinner, J. D. (1998). Mothers determine sexual preferences. *Nature, 395*, 229–230.

Kutchinsky, B. (1976). Deviance and criminality: The case of voyeur in a peeper's paradise. *Diseases of the Nervous System, 37*, 145–151.

Lavin, M. (2008). Voyeurism: Psychopathology and theory. In D. Richard Laws & W. T. O'Donohue (Eds.), *Sexual deviance: Theory, assessment, and treatment* (pp. 305–319). New York, NY: The Guilford Press.

Laws, D. R., & Marshall, W. L. (1990). A conditioning theory of the etiology and maintenance of deviant sexual preference and behavior. In W. L. Marshall & others (Eds.), *Handbook of sexual assault.* New York: Springer Science + Business Media.

Lorand, S., & Schneer, H. (1967). Sexual deviations. In A. Freedman & H. Kaplan (Eds.), *Comprehensive Textbook of Psychiatry* (pp. 977–988). Baltimore: Williams & Wilkins.

Maletzky, B. M., & McGovern, K. B. (1991). *Treating the sexual offender.* Newbury Park: Sage.

Marshall, W. L., & Barbaree, H. E. (1990). An integrated theory of the etiology of sexual offending. In W. L. Marshall, D. R. Laws, & H. E. Barbaree (Eds.), *Handbook of sexual assault: Issues, theories, and treatment of the offender* (pp. 257–271). New York: Springer Science + Business Media.

McConaghy, N. (1970). Subjective and penile plethysmograph responses to aversion therapy for homosexuality: A follow-up study. *British Journal of Psychiatry, 17*, 555–560.

McGuire, R. J., Carlisle, J. M., & Young, B. G. (1964). Sexual deviations as conditioned behaviour: A hypothesis. *Behavior Research and Therapy, 2*(2–4), 185–190.

Money, J. (1986). *Lovemaps: Clinical concepts of sexual/erotic health and pathology, paraphilia, and gender transposition in childhood, adolescence, and maturity.* New York, NY: Irvington.

Nicolosi, A., Laumann, E. O., Glasser, D. B., Moreira, E. D., Jr., Paik, A., & Gingell, C. (2004). Sexual behaviour and sexual dysfunctions after age 40: The global study of sexual attitudes and behaviors. *Adult Urology, 54*(5), 991–997.

Perry, D. G., & Bussey, K. (1979). The social learning theory of sex differences: Imitation is alive and well. *Journal of Personality and Social Psychology, 37*(10), 1699–1712.

Pinkava, V. (1971). Logical models of sexual deviation. *International Journal of Man-Machine Studies, 3,* 351–374.

Pirelli, B., Esben, E., Almås, E., & Weingarten, K. (2015). Sex positive ways of perceiving sexual turn-on patterns Part I—Understanding. *International Journal of Narrative Therapy & Community Work, 1,* 26–37.

Rachman, S., & Hodgson, R. J. (1968). Experimentally-induced "sexual fetishism": Replication and development. *The Psychological Record, 18*(1), 25–27.

Rhodes, G., Simmons, L. W., & Peters, M. (2005). Attractiveness and sexual behavior: Does attractiveness enhance mating success? *Evolution and Human Behavior, 26,* 186–201.

Rosen, R. C., Shapiro, D., & Schwartz, G. (1975). Voluntary control of penile tumescence. *Psychosomatic Medicine, 37*(6), 479–483.

Rye, B. J., & Meaney, G. J. (2007). Voyeurism. *International Journal of Sexual Health, 19*(1), 47–56.

Schwartz, B. J. (1956). An empirical test of two Freudian hypotheses concerning castration anxiety. *Journal of Personality, 24,* 318–327.

Smith, R. S. (1976). Voyeurism: A literature review. *Archives of Sexual Behavior, 5*(6), 585–608.

Smith, C. A., Ireland, T. O., Park, A., Elwyn, L., & Thornberry, T. P. (2011). Intergenerational continuities and discontinuities in intimate partner violence: A two-generational prospective study. *Journal of Interpersonal Violence, 26*(18), 3720–3752.

Snaith, P. (1983). Exhibitionism: A clinical conundrum. *British Journal of Psychiatry, 143*(3), 231–235.

Sperling, M. (1963). Fetishism in children. *The Psychoanalytic Quarterly, 32*(3), 374–392.

Vicedo, M. (2009). The father of ethology and the foster mother of ducks: Konrad Lorenz as an Expert on Motherhood. *Isis, 100*(2), 263–291.

Weinberg, M. S., Williams, C. J., & Calhan, C. (1995). "If the shoe fits…": Exploring male homosexual foot fetishism. *The Journal of Sex Research, 32*(1), 17–27.

CHAPTER 5

Approaches to Treatment

Abstract This chapter describes a variety of approaches that have been used in the treatment of voyeurism, from aversive conditioning, drug therapies, to talking therapies. As most of the literature briefly describes successful single-case studies or larger empirical studies that do not always identify the voyeurs, it is not always clear if there are any particular methods that can be relied on to work with voyeurs.

Keywords Aversive conditioning · Masturbatory reconditioning Covert sensitisation · Assertiveness training

A variety of possible explanations for voyeurism may equally suggest a variety of approaches to provide intervention. As mentioned earlier, in some cases medication has proved useful, based on the idea that voyeurism may be an expression of obsessive–compulsive disorder, and psychoanalytic theories would, and do, suggest extensive psychoanalytic therapy. Mann and colleagues (2008) cite Hanson and Harris (1997) who suggested then that any treatments for voyeurism should be considered experimental, and 10 years later, Mann et al. endorse that view. Given the lack of literature and the uncertainty of the value of any approach outside the limited case reports, this section will provide a flavour of interventions that have been tried (see Mann et al., 2008, for a more comprehensive overview).

S. Duff, *Voyeurism*, https://doi.org/10.1007/978-3-319-97160-5_5

Aversive Conditioning

Learning theories have suggested that voyeurism can be learned, typically because the behaviour is paired with a positive outcome, such as orgasm, or feelings of power. This implies that if voyeurism were to be paired with something negative, and that negative pairing was more powerful (or extinguished the other, positive, paring), voyeurism would reduce. Or, if voyeurism was a learned strategy to successfully satisfy the need for a sexual outlet then if a different, more prosocial, strategy could be learned to achieve sexual satisfaction then this might be chosen in preference to voyeurism. Many of the early therapeutic approaches for voyeurism, and other forms of behaviour that in this period of psychological treatment were considered deviant and harmful (e.g. homosexuality, cross-dressing, exhibitionism), followed these paths.

A common approach during the development of behavioural treatments was to use electric shock (in some research rather than referring to electric shock it was referred to as "faradic aversion conditioning" e.g. Thorpe, Schmidt, & Castell, 1963) as the negative pairing of choice and there are a variety of case studies where people have been shocked, either in reality or in imagination, thinking about viewing or actually viewing stimuli that they found arousing. Such approaches have been variously used in attempts to extinguish fetishism (Bond & Evans, 1967), sadistic fantasies (Mees, 1966), paedophilia (Marshall & Williams, 1975), and homosexuality (Cautela, 1967). Examples where this approach was used with a voyeur is the work of Rangaswamy (1987) and that of Gaupp, Stern, and Ratliff (1971). In the latter case, the client was a 24-year-old man who self-reported voyeurism since the age of 10. At the time of treatment, he was watching college women, with a specific interest in their breasts. His view was that the behaviour was triggered by boredom or frustration. He claimed that there was no sexual element to his voyeurism but the authors write, "the client was not convincing in this regard" (p. 556). He also reported having a satisfactory sex life with his wife. The treatment consisted of being presented with 11 slides that referred to voyeur-related concepts ("masturbating to peeping fantasies", "spying on strange girl's sexual privacy") that were paired with electric shocks that he received on his ankle, for a duration of .3 s. The remaining 11 slides, which were not paired with shocks, related to the triggers for voyeurism ("boredom", "frustration") and triggers that would lead the client to have sex with his wife ("sexual intercourse with W"—it is not clear if W was his wife's name or in the account of the treatment this is used to replace her name for anonymity). The authors recorded the number of self-reported incidents of voyeurism during treatment and report that the urge to "peep", actual "peeping", the urge to masturbate and actual masturbation (presumably to fantasies of "peeping") reduced to zero by the end of 12 weekly sessions. Other approaches using a similar technique include "anticipatory avoidance", whereby once the client has experienced aversive conditioning for a period of time they are able to avoid the shocks if they actively turn off the stimuli that are considered deviant. So, for example, if the deviant pictures are of women, seen through a window, undressing, turning off the display within a given time will prevent the associated shock from occurring. Maletzky and McGovern (1991) provide a brief case example where this approach was used successfully with a voyeur (p. 141). Other case studies report similar successes, either suggesting that such techniques are very useful or that only positive cases are ever reported. As aversive conditioning techniques have almost entirely been replaced the latter explanation is more likely, particularly as some studies have suggested that when used in order to change sexual behaviour there is little evidence of change (e.g. Conrad & Wincze, 1976).

Other forms of aversive conditioning include the use of unpleasant smells as the paired stimulus or shaming therapies (see Marshall & Barbaree, 1978). In one version of shaming therapy, a person acts out their behaviour and then is either neutrally viewed by professionals (Reitz & Keil, 1971; Wickramasekera, 1972) or mocked by professionals. The latter is a risky approach as it might anger the client, rather than acting as a negative reinforcer to the behaviour under treatment, and this might lead to aggressive outbursts against professionals. A second form of shaming therapy is based on working with clients who are already ashamed of their behaviour and are asked to carry it out (or, a close imitation of it) in front of professionals. The idea is that this increases their own feelings of shame and acts as an aversive outcome. Serber (1970) provides a very brief account of some case studies, one of whom was a voyeur. In that situation, the voyeur was asked to observe someone undressing through a one-way mirror. Serber reports that after 3 sessions of this form of shaming the man, who had been a voyeur for 15 years with a frequency of voyeurism of once or twice a month, only reported one re-enactment in the next 6 months. The other cases involve transvestism, paedophilia, exhibitionism, and frotteurism, and all of the results are similarly positive. Some therapists have been more inventive in the unpleasant ways that they have treated their clients, although there are no reports of these more extreme approaches with voyeurs. For example, Quinn, Harbisan, and McAllister (1970) describe that a homosexual man, who was deprived of water, was given sips of lime juice if he became aroused to pictures of naked women.

Masturbatory Reconditioning

Masturbatory reconditioning is another approach that has been described and used in attempts to change sexual behaviour. One version of this is that gradually one replaces the deviant stimuli viewed during masturbation and at orgasm (for example, pictures of a naked woman through a window) with non-deviant stimuli (pictures of a naked woman). Initially, the orgasm will "accidentally" occur when the non-deviant picture is presented, if the timing is right, and gradually the idea is that this picture is brought in earlier and earlier in the process, training the individual to be able to masturbate and orgasm to non-deviant stimuli. A second approach that is also referred to as masturbatory reconditioning is satiation treatment. Here, the client is asked to repeatedly masturbate to their preferred, deviant stimuli, with the idea that eventually it becomes painful and unpleasant, and as such the idea of becoming aroused to these kinds of stimuli is linked to a strong negative outcome (see Konopacki and Oei, 1988, for a case study). Jackson (1969) reported using a form of masturbatory reconditioning, known as directed masturbation, with a voyeur. The man was told to use non-voyeuristic pictures of heterosexual behaviour for masturbation for two weeks and then to use pictures of naked females for the following two weeks. Jackson reports that nine months later the client had not engaged in voyeurism. Again this is a technique that appears to have lost favour. Laws and Marshall (1991) wrote, "The masturbatory reconditioning literature is remarkable more for the enthusiasm it has produced in clinicians than for the empirical support it can offer for the efficacy of the techniques" (p. 14).

Covert Sensitisation

Covert sensitisation is a process whereby an individual imagines taking part in some form of behaviour, and then imagines negative consequences, with the aim of reducing fantasies and behaviours that are the potential precursors to offending behaviour. As in example, we could ask a person who loiters outside schools to watch children to imagine herself walking up to a school playground and stopping and then to imagine feeling a hand on their shoulder and seeing a police officer, who then proceeds to arrest her and take her to the police cells. Some authors report pairing this negative fantasy with a strong, unpleasant smell to make the whole experience more negative (e.g. Maletzky, 1991). Lamontagne and Lesage (1986) provide an example of this technique with an exhibitionist; the man was asked to imagine that he exposed himself and then imagine that his victim would react angrily and reprimand him or to imagine that his wife would leave him. Hawton (1983) provides a case study of a voyeur where covert sensitisation was used as part of his treatment. The man's voyeurism seemed to be triggered when he went out drinking with friends and this was managed by asking him to go home and masturbate rather than to go to the local nurses home to watch the student nurses. However, once this was no longer an issue the client mentioned that he was starting to have voyeuristic thoughts during the day. Hawton writes, "He therefore started to practise covert sensitization when these thoughts arose, using the image of his being caught and ridiculed by a group of girls as the aversive thought" (p. 252).

Assertiveness Training

One explanation for sexual offending, in some cases, is that individuals do not have a good understanding of the societal norms for achieving their goals, or they are afraid of trying to achieve what are considered normal societal goals (such as being in a relationship, having sex). The idea of assertiveness training is to provide people with the necessary knowledge, skills, and resilience to overcome these gaps in their knowledge and their fears so that they do not have to resort to antisocial means to be successful. There are descriptions of the use of assertiveness training with sexual offenders (Gilmour, McCormick, & de Ruiter, 1981), and Maletzky and McGovern (1991) provide a brief description of its use with a voyeur, where it was applied after successful use of aversion techniques. From Maletzky and McGovern's description, it is not clear if this was considered an integral part of the offence-focussed work or an additional phase because the man had "become more introverted as therapy progressed" (p. 152). Similarly, how success was measured is not provided, in relation to change in offending, but rather, "within several months, [he] was dating an attractive woman and had asked for, and received, a raise" (p. 152). These authors provide a second case study, which again could be understood as assertiveness training, with a voyeur of 16 who had very limited experience with females. He was given a variety of homework tasks to speak to females of his own age, gradually increasing the level of risk he was taking (such as giving compliments, asking someone on a date), and this was reported as successful. This kind of in vivo intervention may result in a secondary benefit; if the interactions with people are positive, that can act as a reinforcer, making the prosocial behaviour more likely to reoccur and increasing the individual's self-esteem (see Maletzky and McGovern, 1991, p. 125). Of course, there is always the potential for interactions not to have gone as hoped, so it is important that people are provided with suitable exit strategies and resilience to cope with such situations.

Drug Therapy

The premise of drug therapy is that sexual offending can be managed by reducing an individual's interest in or ability to have sex by using antiandrogens (chemical castration) and serotonin reuptake inhibitors. This is an evolution of the idea of surgical castration where the removal of the testicles would reduce the amount of testosterone in the blood stream and thus reduce sexual drive. There are positive reports of the reduction of sexual recidivism due to surgical castration (Heim & Hursch, 1979), although it would be interesting to examine if there are changes in other forms of antisocial behaviour after castration, either because the sexual drive has been removed (which may not be the actual cause of offending behaviour) or due to associated side effects. Chemical castration of men with prostate cancer has demonstrated that there is an associated increase in anxiety and depression (Almeida, Waterreus, Spry, Flicker, & Martins, 2004), so it is plausible that some side effects may impact negatively on the behaviour of vulnerable individuals.

Abouesh and Clayton (1999) have described a case of voyeurism that was treated with paroxetine as do Sidi and Midin (2008), where the use of the drug was also combined with aversion therapy. In this latter case, the authors report that their client, who filmed his sisters-in-law in the shower, would become sexually aroused at the sound of the shower and would become anxious in his efforts to stop himself turning on the camera that he had secretly installed in the bathroom. He reported that he was frustrated with his inability to control his behaviour. In addition to his voyeuristic behaviour, he would collect and categorise any hair and nail clippings that he could find once the women had left the bathroom. The use of paroxetine appears to be because his voyeurism was believed to be obsessional and the treatment is reported as having been successful, with no self-reported reoccurrence since treatment.

Saleh and Berlin (2003) provide an overview of drug treatments for people with a variety of paraphilias. A problem with this review and with other original research is that either a range of paraphilias is included in the work (e.g. Coleman, Cesnik, Moore, & Dwyer, 1992; Koo et al., 2013) or voyeurs are not included, so it is difficult to know what specific treatments have been used and might have been successful with voyeurs. For example, Bradford and Pawlak (1993) describe the use of cyproterone acetate as an antiandrogen with 19 paraphilic men. None of these are identified as voyeurs. Certainly, the research appears to be positive and research is ongoing, particularly with regard to individuals who sexually assault children and rapists (for a review see Lewis, Grubin, Ross, & Das, 2017).

Talking Therapy

There are surprisingly few examples of talking therapies with voyeurs, as previously identified by Mann et al. (2008). Despite the lack of evidence for CBT, they suggest a five-step approach that, based on their clinical experience, may be useful, consisting of (i) examining the client's sexual and attachment experiences, (ii) considering the client's sexual knowledge, (iii) exploring the client's beliefs about sexual and intimacy behaviours, (iv) discussing the client's sexual interests, and (v) developing relapse prevention plans. Given that such a treatment plan has been specified by the experts in the field, it would be useful to have it tested with a clinical population with the aim of developing intervention guidelines for voyeurs.

The dearth of evidence for talking therapies may be for a variety of reasons. Primarily it may be that in many therapeutic regimes voyeurs are grouped together with other sexual offenders and so there is little specific information on the impact of CBT or any particular ways of working with these people. Linked to this is the issue that there may be relatively few voyeurs who, despite being convicted, come to the attention of professionals; they may not be required to have assessments or to receive some form of intervention as a part of their sentence. It may also be that voyeurism is not considered of enough concern that it requires our attention. It is difficult to identify what the reasons may be, but it is clear that the issue of voyeurism is not central. For example, Brown's (2005) book on treating sex offenders does not mention voyeurs, nor do Stinson and Becker (2013), or Marshall, Fernandez, Marshall, and Serran, (2006).

Kleinplatz (2014) provides a case study of a voyeur that she worked with using experiential psychotherapy. In this approach, rather than working with voyeurism as a problem the idea is to use it as an opportunity to explore individuals' strong feelings and use those as a focus for personality change. In Kleinplatz's example it appears that the voyeurism is linked to concerns of being ignored and abandoned as a child and that these feelings prevented the client from expressing and experiencing his adult sexuality. One this was identified and "Jeff" found ways, in collaboration with his wife, to be more expressive and adventurous his feelings changed, his sexual behaviour and experiences changed, and he no longer engaged in voyeurism.

The variety of treatment options and theories are not founded on a large database of research, but rather through case studies, and forming hypotheses with what has worked in understanding and treating other forms of sexual offending. Ideally we would investigate voyeurs more systematically, both those who have been identified through the criminal justice system and those who self-identify, to better understand them and their behaviour. Using this knowledge, we would have a greater facility for developing interventions. That may be the best way to progress. However, the next best method is to consider a case in great detail, through the process of assessment, formulation, and treatment, and then follow that person for a period of time post-treatment. That is the approach taken here and the next section focuses on KS, the case study.

References

Abouesh, A., & Clayton, A. (1999). Compulsive voyeurism and exhibitionism: A clinical response to paroxetine. *Archives of Sexual Behavior, 28*(1), 23–30.

Almeida, O. P., Waterreus, A., Spry, N., Flicker, L., & Martins, R. N. (2004). One year follow-up study of the association between chemical castration, sex hormones, beta-amyloid, memory and depression in men. *Psychoneuroendocrinology, 29*(8), 1071–1081.

Bond, I. K., & Evans, D. R. (1967). Avoidance therapy: Its use in two cases of underwear fetishism. *Canadian Medical Association Journal, 96*(16), 1160–1162.

Bradford, J. M. W., & Pawlak, A. (1993). Double-blind placebo crossover study of cyproterone acetate in the treatment of the paraphilias. *Archives of Sexual Behavior, 22*(5), 383–402.

Brown, S. (2005). *Treating sex offenders: An introduction to sex offender treatment programmes.* Cullompton, Devon: Willan Publishing.

Cautela, J. R. (1967). Covert sensitization. *Psychological Reports, 20*(2), 459–468.

Coleman, E., Cesnik, J., Moore, A.-M., & Dwyer, M. (1992). An exploratory study of the role of psychotropic medications in the treatment of sex offenders. *Journal of Offender Rehabilitation, 18*(3–4), 75–88.

Conrad, S., & Wincze, J. (1976). Orgasmic reconditioning: A controlled study of its effects upon the sexual arousal and behavior of male homosexuals. *Behavior Therapy, 7,* 155–166.

Gaupp, L. A., Stern, R. M., & Ratliff, R. G. (1971). The use of aversion-relief procedures in the treatment of a case of voyeurism. *Behavior Therapy, 2,* 585–588.

Gilmour, D. R., McCormick, I. A., & de Ruiter, C. A. (1981). Group assertion training for adult male offenders: Internal validity. *Behavior Therapy, 12,* 274–279.

Hawton, K. (1983). Behavioural approaches to the management of sexual deviations. *British Journal of Psychiatry, 143*(3), 248–255.

Heim, N., & Hursch, C. J. (1979). Castration for sexual offenders: Treatment or punishment? A review and critique of recent European literature. *Archives of Sexual Behavior, 8,* 281–304.

Jackson, B. T. (1969). A case study of voyeurism treated by counterconditioning. *Behavioral Research & Therapy, 7,* 133–134.

Kleinplatz, P. J. (2014). The paraphilias: An experiential approach to "dangerous" desires. In Y. M. Binik & K. S. K. Hall (Eds.), *Principles and practice of sex therapy* (5th ed., pp. 195–218). New York, NY: Guilford.

Konopacki, W. P., & Oei, T. P. S. (1988). Interruption in the maintenance of compulsive sexual disorder: Two case studies. *Archives of Sexual Behavior, 17,* 411–419.

Koo, K. C., Shim, G. S., Park, H. H., Rha, K. H., Choi, Y. D., Chung, B. H., et al. (2013). Treatment outcomes of chemical castration on Korean sex offenders. *Journal of Forensic and Legal Medicine, 20,* 563–566.

Lamontagne, Y., & Lesage, A. (1986). Private exposure and covert sensitization in the treatment of exhibitionism. *Journal of Behavior Therapy and Experimental Psychiatry, 17,* 197–201.

Laws, D. R., & Marshall, W. L. (1991). Masturbatory reconditioning of sexual deviates: An evaluative review. *Advances in Behavior Research and Therapy, 13*(1), 13–25.

Lewis, A., Grubin, D., Ross, C. C., & Das, M. (2017). Gonadotrophin-releasing hormone agonist treatment for sexual offenders: A systematic review. *Journal of Psychopharmacology, 31*(10), 1281–1293.

Maletzky, B. M. (1991). *Treating the Sexual Offender*. Thousand Oaks, CA: Sage.

Maletzky, B. M., & McGovern, K. B. (1991). *Treating the sexual offender*. Newbury Park: Sage.

Mann, R. E., Ainsworth, F., Al-Attar, Z., & Davies, M. (2008). Voyeurism: Assessment and treatment. In D. R. Laws & W. T. O'Donohue (Eds.), *Sexual Deviance* (2nd ed., pp. 320–335). New York: Guilford Press.

Marshall, W. L., & Barbaree, H. E. (1978). The reduction of deviant arousal: Satiation treatment for sexual aggressors. *Criminal Justice and Behaviour, 5*(4), 294–303.

Marshall, W. L., Fernandez, Y. M., Marshall, L. E., & Serran, G. A. (Eds.). (2006). *Sexual offender treatment: Controversial issues*. Hoboken, NJ: Wiley.

Marshall, W. L., & Williams, S. M. (1975). *A behavioral treatment program for incarcerated sex offenders: Some tentative results*. Paper presented at the Annual Meeting of the Association for the Advancement of Behavior Therapy, San Francisco, December.

Mees, H. L. (1966). Sadistic fantasies modified by aversive conditioning and substitution: A case study. *Behaviour Research and Therapy, 4*(4), 317–320.

Quinn, J. T., Harbisan, J. J., & McAllister, H. (1970). An attempt to shape human penile responses. *Behavior Research and Therapy, 8*, 213–216.

Rangaswamy, K. (1987). Treatment of voyeurism by behavior therapy. *Child Psychiatry Quarterly, 20*, 381–386.

Reitz, W. E., & Keil, W. E. (1971). Behavioral treatment of an exhibitionist. *Journal of Behavior Therapy and Experimental Psychiatry, 2*(1), 67–69.

Saleh, F. M., & Berlin, F. (2003). Sex hormones, neurotransmitters, and psychopharmacological treatments in men with paraphilic disorders. *Journal of Child Sexual Abuse, 12*(3–4), 233–253.

Serber, M. (1970). Shame aversion therapy. *Journal of Behavioral Therapy and Experimental Psychiatry, 1*, 213–215.

Sidi, H., & Midin, M. (2008). Voyeurism with sexual fantasy on female body parts: A subtype of obsessive-compulsive disorder? *Malaysian Journal of Psychiatry Ejournal, 17*(1), 1–6.

Stinson, J. D., & Becker, J. V. (2013). *Treating sex offenders: An evidence-based manual*. New York, NY: The Guildford Press.

Thorpe, J. G., Schmidt, E., & Castell, D. (1963). A comparison of positive and negative (aversive) conditioning in the treatment of homosexuality. *Behaviour Research and Therapy, 1*(2–4), 357–362.

Wickramasekera, I. (1972). A technique for controlling a certain type of sexual exhibitionism. *Psychotherapy: Theory, Research and Practice, 9*(3), 207–210.

CHAPTER 6

The Case Study: KS

Abstract This chapter presents KS, the case study, along with the detailed assessment of his offending behaviour and all aspects of his life, including his early experiences and his relationship history.

Keywords Psychometric tests for voyeurism · Frotteurism
Iconophilia · Upskirting

For the purposes of this case study, we will identify the male in question as KS. To reassure readers KS did provide informed consent to be a case study for academic purposes and this consent has been seen by the publishers. He was also informed of the regulations related to confidentiality and the consequences of disclosing further offences. Case studies of voyeurism are not unprecedented, although noticeably rare, and other examples that may be of interest are those provided by Jackson (1969), Gaupp, Stern, and Ratliff (1971), Nelson (1977), and Abouesh and Clayton (1999), amongst others, although the vast majority are short case reports. For brevity, along with the material that was gained through assessment, some of the thinking that resulted, prior to the development of a formulation, will also be presented, in this section.

As clinicians will be well aware, working with people in the areas of sexual behaviour is difficult due to a number of factors such as secrecy, fear, shame, embarrassment, each potentially impacting on the honesty with which an individual will approach assessment and treatment. Even

S. Duff, *Voyeurism*, https://doi.org/10.1007/978-3-319-97160-5_6

where there are other sources of evidence we know that individuals may lie at different times to different people, individuals may forget details and make up information to maintain a coherent narrative, and errors do occur in official records. Ultimately, we rely on developing a good relationship with our clients, in a safe environment, where the rules of confidentiality and conduct are explicit, and professional boundaries are maintained, abiding by the ethical regulations of our governing bodies. We work collaboratively to form a shared understanding and a shared solution. We then believe that when a client expresses a wish to change, they will also feel able to be open and honest. With KS, particularly given his unsuccessful prior engagement with services (see below), great pains were taken to develop and maintain rapport throughout and where accounts differed in our sessions and data available from other professionals he was appropriately challenged. As such, the information presented below, directly from KS, is presented as accurate. Some details irrelevant to the assessment and intervention have been changed to preserve KS' anonymity.

An important caveat with this case study, and one that might be employed by any critically engaged reader of case studies, is that it presents a particular type of voyeur. As we will see, KS did not deny his behaviour, nor did he present it as opportunistic, or part of a more general healthy sexual life. It was not part of sexual courtship nor an element of other offending, such as contact offending, and it does not appear that he had other paraphilias (certainly if he did they had not led to him being arrested and convicted). As such we might refer to him, in terms Lavin (2008) used, as a "full-fledged voyeur" rather than "simply a creepy opportunist" (p. 316). This is important because not all voyeurs who are referred for assessment and treatment will be like KS in their behaviour and in their presentation—reflective, educated, intelligent, and hoping to change.

It is also important to understand something of the therapeutic setting. The service that KS was referred to is a specialist community service that is known for a focus on sexual offenders. Predominantly we work with men who have offended against children, using a variety of group and one-to-one interventions including eye movement desensitisation and reprocessing (EMDR), schema therapy, mindfulness, cognitive analytic therapy (CAT), and cognitive behavioural therapy (CBT). As a community service, despite out specialism, we receive referrals that cover a wide range of offences, with a wide range of mental health, personality, and intellectual challenges and as such our approach and experience is broad-based and ideographic. Although the work and the inferences drawn from working with KS will be presented as mine (in collaboration with KS), this is not to deny to huge value that supervision and discussion with colleagues offered in considering KS and his circumstances.

Offending Behaviour

KS' first conviction occurred in 2001 when he was caught inside female toilets. His view was that after being convicted, he stopped offending due to lack of opportunity rather than because he had any less interest. He reported that he was aware that he "needed help" at that time as his behaviour was having obvious negative consequences, but he was unaware of what help might be available, how to access support, and was too embarrassed to seek advice from his GP. His second conviction occurred in 2007 for seven offences of voyeurism and attempted voyeurism. His third conviction occurred in 2012. On this occasion, he reported that he was in a pub drinking and feeling low, and noticed, when he went outside to the pub garden to smoke, that the window to the female toilets faced into the garden. He waited until he saw a woman enter the toilet and held his mobile telephone through the open window of the toilet to film the woman. On a subsequent occasion of doing this, a victim saw the telephone and took it out of his hand and alerted the police. The police found evidence of upskirting pictures on his telephone and PC.

Assessment

At the time that KS was assessed and intervention was carried out, he was in his early 40s. He is a white, single, heterosexual male, with a university education in a numerate subject, and is clearly intelligent, thoughtful, and reflective, and during our work it was evident he was trying to understand his behaviour and seek explanations, triggers, and the protective factors related to it. It was also evident that his behaviour was not just causing him legal problems but was having an impact on how he felt about himself and about his future. For example, he stated that in his view if he were convicted again he would likely receive a prison sentence of the order of 10 years. He was not embarrassed by his behaviour, so his desire to change was not driven by shame, rather a real sense that without change his life was unlikely to develop in the ways that he hoped.

KS' first conviction occurred in his late 20s when he was reported for being in female toilets. He was later convicted for both voyeurism linked to attempts (some successful) to see, hear, and record women in toilets, both from inside the cubicles and from outside windows, and for taking pictures and videos up women's skirts, the last of which occurred in his late 30s. For his last offence, KS received 6 months' imprisonment, suspended for two years, hours of community service in three figures, and the requirement to sign the sex offender register for seven years. KS had undergone 2 separate rounds of the National Probation Service's Sex Offender Treatment Programme (Northumbria Sex Offender Group Programme—NSOGP), once in 2009 and again in 2014. These were considered unsuccessful because he had gone on to reoffend, at which point he was referred to a specialist NHS community forensic service. At this point, he reported to his probation officer, his police liaison officer, and to the community service that he was keen to access support to make positive changes to his life, which he saw as specifically related to his offending.

There was no evidence from KS' records or from his own accounts of his behaviour that his offending had escalated over time (beyond his index offences), either in his fantasies, planning, or his offending. He harboured no interest in committing burglary to access women's underwear, to assault women, or to carry out any form of contact offence. Since his last conviction, he reported at the assessment that he was managing to restrict his voyeuristic behaviour to watching online pornography that fitted with his two areas of interest—women using the toilet (here referred to as *urolagnia*) and upskirting, whilst also being aware of what he had identified as potential triggers. Despite an awareness of these triggers, he did not consistently choose to act to keep himself safe. For example, KS identified that alcohol was a potential trigger for offence-supportive thoughts yet he would regularly decide to watch football games in a local pub and drink; the amount he drank dictated purely by how much money he had available. Some of his previous offending directly followed time spent drinking and then, on his way home, starting to feel low, resulting in him entering other pubs or clubs and attempting to access women's toilets. Additionally, he would become distracted if he saw a woman enter public toilets yet whilst in a pub to watch a football match he would choose a seat that gave him both a good view of the television screen and of the door to the women's toilets. He reported that he considered he was hypervigilant to the movement of women in pubs and clubs, if they appeared to be going towards the toilets.

KS also stated that he did not exhibit any other problematic behaviours or have thoughts linked to other paraphilias that have been frequently associated with voyeurism. For example, he had never exposed himself, sexually assaulted or raped anyone, rubbed against people for sexual reasons, behaved in sadistic ways, or had sexual thoughts about children. His sexual activities, outside of his offending behaviour and related pornography use, were directed at adult, consenting peers, and within these relationships there was no evidence of, for example, fetishism. There was no evidence of thoughts to harm himself or other people.

At the assessment, KS was not in a relationship and had not been for approximately 20 years. Overall he described living in relative isolation. In part this was through concerns that his convictions had been reported in the media, accompanied by photographs, and he was wary of being recognised as he continued to live in the same area. This had resulted in him disengaging with peers. KS also reported that he did not feel socially confident or competent and raised concerns about his sexual knowledge and performance. He had no other prior convictions or warnings on record.

Early History

KS reported that he was brought up by his mother and her parents for the first 10 years of his life. He described himself as quite a shy child. His grandfather died when KS was 10 years old, his grandmother when he was 16 years old. At no point during his childhood does he recall there being a father figure in his life or that his mother engaged in any intimate relationships. He reports having had positive relationships with his grandparents and with his mother, which continues to this day. The notable element of KS' early life is that, by his description, it was unremarkable. He reported no traumatic events, no bullying, no unwanted sexual experiences, and progression through school appeared to be routine. He described no sense that his mother or grandparents had particular views of sex or women and suggests that he grew up in what he referred to as a sexually neutral environment. By that he meant that there were no discussions of sex and that there were no obvious elements of sexual discrimination or roles based on gender. The absence of his father, the death of his grandparents, and all other life stages he described without any evidence of reactions that raised concerns.

One feature that did stand out, although not to KS, was that he recalled that throughout his childhood his mother would use the toilet without closing the door and he remembers frequently seeing this. KS reported no feelings of sexual arousal to seeing his mother use the toilet, or any sense that she intended this to be sexual. As has been considered in a variety of explanations of voyeurism presented above, such an early experience, although not recognised as sexual by KS, may have been an important factor for the development of voyeurism.

Education

KS described his education as uneventful. He was successful enough to be accepted to university although there he reported that he did not focus on his studies in his final year and graduated with a lower class degree. He was unable to describe any particular academic difficulties, truanting, or problems with being bullied, rather just becoming disillusioned with his area of study and spending more time socialising than studying.

Employment

Despite his university degree, KS has not worked within the profession he studied for, nor has he worked in any other professional capacity. All of his jobs have been relatively short term in nature and unskilled. More recently, this has been, by his account, due to the nature of his offending history and not wanting to divulge his criminal record, which has restricted him to finding agency work. As such, he has worked mostly in factories and on building sites. Whilst he was offending, the nature of his employment did not work well as a protective factor as he did not find it intellectually demanding and due to his shyness he did not develop a peer group, so outside of his work hours there were no secondary gains to employment. However, during the time at work, he was engaged and reports no thoughts of offending. His wages allowed him to afford cannabis and to drink, and to have access to the Internet and his evenings were mostly spent alone and he would access the Internet to entertain himself. The nature of his work was also somewhat intermittent, meaning there were periods when he had more time away from work and less money, both of which impacted on his mood and the opportunity to find antisocial methods to use his time. Often he would fill this time with walking around town with an eye to capturing upskirt images or at home using the Internet to watch pornography.

Substance Use

At the university, KS began to use alcohol and cannabis, but he reports no other drug use at that time. Both were used in social settings initially, when KS was in an environment that supported relatively easy socialisation. His alcohol use would not have been considered problematic given his age and the setting, and he reported that it did not impact on his academic abilities. He was unable to identify any negative effects of cannabis use although stated that he would smoke most evenings. KS reported that after university both alcohol and cannabis took on more of a problematic role in that they were both used as a form of self-medication to manage feelings of isolation and a lack of employment. As a keen football supporter, he would often go to the local pub to watch away games and rely on consumption of alcohol to manage the fact that he was on his own. Often he would drink to excess and ruminate on what he considered the negative aspects of his life (lack of job, money, and girlfriend) and this, as reported by KS, would frequently result in him distracting himself by watching women in the pub go to the toilet and thinking about what they might be doing. In a similar fashion, he reported that when at home he would use cannabis and when disinhibited would frequently access online pornography, particularly of a voyeuristic type.

Early Sexual Behaviour and Relationships

KS reported no identifiable events of a traumatic sexual nature and appears to have developed a sexual interest in females around puberty. He was able to describe that he and his male friends would discuss sex, often, in his view, people dishonestly bragging about their knowledge and experience of sex. A factor that is useful to consider here is that, to some extent, KS had more opportunity than some of his peers to have a degree of knowledge of females given that he had routinely seen his mother use the toilet and (see below) had already developed a curiosity in females going to the toilet. There were no early sexual encounters directly, although a number of events that took on something of an erotic nature for KS (see below).

According to Probation reports, KS described that he had had a number of intimate relationships, some of which were one-night stands, the first that included sexual intercourse occurring when he was 17 years of age. He said that his longest relationship was 3 months and that his final relationship ended when he was 23 years of age. KS reported no concerns at that time with the sexual element of his relationships and considered that his behaviour was typical and appropriate. With regard to his dating behaviour, KS stated that he is not one for direct approaches, as he believes that he has a tendency towards being awkward. However, his strategy has proven successful, although he does report that usually this relies on substance use on his part so that he is less self-conscious. When he was involved in relationships, he had a fear of those relationships ending, resulting in behaviour that has had him labelled, according to his description, as "too clingy".

At the time of reporting to Probation, he claimed that lack of relationships was due to poor finances and little time. However, the true underlying reason became apparent during the assessment, and this appeared entirely due to the way that his final relationship ended. As far as KS was concerned, the relationship was progressing well and he was unaware of any issues that his then partner might have had with him. However, with no prior warning she was very disparaging regarding his sexual knowledge and abilities, indicating that in her view he should know more and be doing more. He was not informed as to the exact nature of what she was expecting from him (i.e. was it a lack of particular behaviours or a perceived lack of skill in behaviours) and he was engaging in all of the sexual behaviours that he was then familiar with (manual masturbation, oral sex, sexual intercourse). Although this event had occurred nearly 20 years previously, he remained uncomfortable discussing it and reported ongoing feelings of inadequacy in knowledge and performance; he was convinced that he would now not be able to sexually satisfy anyone and that people would know from his particular repertoire of skills that he had not, in his opinion, developed sexual experience commensurate with his age and the experience that people would assume of a man in his early 40s. For these reasons, he was no longer seeking intimate relationships with women and, on the occasions when a woman had initiated sexual contact with him, he had made excuses to prevent any sexual activity. One example he gave was that having met a woman at a club and her having invited him home and to her bed, he was able to kiss her but when she attempted to progress to genital contact he said he was too drunk and tired to continue. He spent the night and left early the next morning.

KS specifically reported that in his relationships he does not want to know what his partner's underwear are like, how she urinates, or to have her urinate for him, and he had never attempted to listen to, view, or film any of his partners. It is plausible that this may be in part due to the fact that all of his relationships have been brief. However, on the face of it this suggests that either relationships fulfil the needs that he otherwise meets through urolagnia and upskirting or that despite wanting to engage in these behaviours he does not have the confidence to discuss it with his partners. However, of interest is that whilst in a relationship he finds that sexual thoughts that do not involve *urolagnia* or upskirting can be equally sexually arousing and satisfying, and can still be used for masturbation.

It is likely that KS' concerns are compounded by his use of pornography which routinely shows sexual intimacy as highly satisfying for both partners, where the people involved are portrayed as having perfect bodies, perfect technique, and being creative and widely knowledgeable. That he has spent more time viewing pornography than being involved in relationships could result in him believing that this is the level of knowledge and expertise (and satisfaction) that is expected and is routine in relationships, thus highlighting further his lack of experience and knowledge.

KS had done nothing to try to deal with his perceived lack of knowledge or skills and also perceived them as more generally inhibiting him socially. Although the Internet and various books and magazines offer a wealth of sexual information and social opportunities he had not sought out that information, he did not appear to try to engage in conversations about sex with his few male friends, and he had not tried to gain practical experience (although he has made use of prostitutes as outlined below). The extent to which this lack of proactivity is something peculiar to KS is not clear; it is entirely possible that men who feel ill-informed (or have been told that they are lacking in some way) about sexual matters do not routinely find ways to educate themselves. It is also not clear the extent to which this may be a risk factor. What is clear is that we need to consider the ways in which people are able to seek support and education regarding sexual behaviour and to examine how it may play a role in quality of life and concerning behaviours. Research with people with intellectual disabilities has suggested that poorer sexual knowledge does not appear to be a risk factor with this population (Talbot & Langdon, 2006) nor do educational problems appear to be linked to paedophilia in sexual offenders (Bogaert, 2001).

Urolagnia

KS was able to recount a number of events that he perceived as potentially linked to his offending behaviour. When he was approximately 9 years old, he remembers working in a potato field and adult women urinating in the field and him finding this "interesting". He was unable to provide any further detail as to what it was that was interesting or how this made him feel at the time. He also recalls that before starting secondary school he was attending a school open day with his mother, a friend, his friend's mother and his friend's sister, the latter needing to urinate and doing so in an alleyway. KS recalled her mother saying to her "do you have to do it like that?" and wanting to see. His view is this might have been his first sexualised or "curious" experience related to *urolagnia* potentially because she was "doing something different", which suggested to him that different women may act differently.

KS identified in sessions that regular arousal to females urinating began around the age of 11 when he was with friends and one of his female friends went behind a bush to urinate. KS was unable to identify what he might have been thinking and feeling at the time of this event, but reflecting back he suggested that it was because he was aware that the girl would be partially undressed, that he wondered how she would be positioned to urinate (squatting, leaning against a tree), and that it was clearly a secret act because she had hidden herself from the group of friends. In parallel with these events, KS stated that conversations with friends at school were beginning to focus on the anatomical differences between boys and girls and on issues of sex; thus, there was an additional source of curiosity for him.

In contrast to the above, a Probation report states that KS recalled at school, at 16 years of age, first discovering that he became sexually aroused to the sound of a female urinating, which he heard by chance. At school he was known for having looked over the stalls at girls and gained the nickname "Peeping Tom". At this early stage, he became aware of the consequences of his actions and reported that he was then concerned about who might know of his behaviour. Despite these consequences impacting on how he was perceived by his peers, this was not powerful enough to prevent his behaviour, although he became more surreptitious and opportunistic. He recounted having been at a café and waiting to use the communal public toilet and knowing that a woman had gone in before him and that he made great efforts to hear her, without being noticed. His view is that he had not intentionally followed the woman to the toilet, knowing that it was a single, unisex toilet, but that he took advantage of the situation. Around this same time KS reported that at a house party he purposefully walked in on a woman when he knew that she was using the toilet, and that his motivation was solely to see how she used the toilet.

Despite some confusion as to the start of his sexual interest in women using the toilet—based on the nature of our relationship and that he divulged his earlier response after some time working with me I am inclined to accept the earlier starting point—it is clear that KS had developed an ongoing interest in women using the toilet and that it incorporated a sexual element. The idea of females urinating became an element of his sexual fantasy life and masturbation. KS remembers becoming aroused when watching a detective series on television and a female character was portrayed as going to the toilet, thus this generalised from women that he had opportunistically seen going into a toilet, or had urinated in his vicinity, to third-party descriptions of women using the toilet.

Although he recognises that he had developed a curiosity and potential sexual response to the idea of females urinating, KS stated that whilst in 6th form and at the university he did not offend, possibly because of having a high workload and because there were opportunities for consensual, contact sexual experiences. Indeed, he reported that he did fantasise during this period but did not attempt to enact his fantasies. This is useful as it suggests that at this stage *urolagnia* was not a major factor in his life, but perhaps an interest that he would become aware of when not occupied with other tasks and/or when there were fewer available sexual outlets. This was borne out by KS revealing that at times when he had less work he was more likely to fantasise. For example, whilst taking an extra year at the university and with less to occupy his time, and with a smaller social group, he would spend time in the bathroom in his house with the hope of seeing the neighbouring women in their bathroom (as the windows were opposite one another). KS was also aware that he was fearful if he were caught and what people might say.

It was not until he was approximately 27 years of age that he began acting on his thoughts and fantasies with an increasing focus on, and efforts to succeed in, seeing women urinating. This he achieved by identifying toilets within university buildings, after he had graduated, that he felt he knew well and where he was able to secrete himself into a cubicle and listen to women, in relative safety. His recollection is that he would become aroused whilst listening to or watching a woman use the toilet. As his *urolagnia* developed, he would, on occasions, make attempts to see or film women urinating. Despite recognising that this increased his chances of being caught, his motivation was both to be able to see how women actually behaved but also that he had developed an opinion of what would be the perfect example of a woman urinating, consisting of her stance, where her clothes were, amongst other factors. This led to a description of his attention to detail, wanting to know the "how"—does a woman sit, squat, undress, how she wipes, her body position. He was of the view that for him there was a "perfect" pose and process, which was not clearly describable. He also reported that the sound was important and that for him it conveyed meaning. For example, a greater sound implied a greater height of squat and the greater the height of the squat, the more the woman might be exposing herself.

Despite being unable to describe the perfect pose, KS was able to describe a hierarchy of features at the top of which is that woman would be squatting. It was suggested to KS that by believing that there was an attainable perfection, this allowed him to continue with his voyeurism until he experienced this perfection. However, without knowing what it consisted of he was unlikely to experience it and so could persuade himself that he needed to continue. Although KS was unable to identify that this was how he thought at the time of his offending, he thought it was a plausible explanation.

On a number of occasions (and see below in relation to upskirting), KS mentioned elements of secrecy as being one of the factors that made his behaviour exciting. His description of this secretive element as "a bloke would never know what goes on in a women's toilet". However, secrecy was not always central to his behaviour. He reported that he has paid approximately 10 prostitutes to urinate for him. He did not tell them how to behave, but had specific preferences regarding how they would squat, the placement of their hands, their head position. He viewed them from the side, rather than trying to get a frontal view of genitals and did not try to physically interact with the women.

An important consideration for this lack of need for secrecy is that although secrecy is important to not get caught, it may be related to a degree of "safety". This may be both in relation to the unusual nature of his preferences and that there is no social interplay (at which he feels awkward and in relation to sex feels unknowledgeable). In a situation where he is completely in control of the interaction and feels that he cannot be judged, it may be that he feels safe enough to be known, to some degree. His viewing behaviour with the prostitutes parallels his offending as he has not expressed an interest in seeing the women's genitals, although has watched voyeuristic pornography that is more direct and he finds that sexually interesting too. This dichotomy is interesting; in real life there is little enthusiasm for direct sight of a woman's genitals, but there is when viewed via pornography. Why might this difference exist? One possibility is that KS has little choice in what pornography offers and the kind that he has an interest in may always include genitals. It is also plausible that, beyond a certain level of intimacy, sex in real life is threatening because one fears that one's lack of knowledge may be exposed. However, when watching pornography there are no reasons to include in one's consequent fantasies any shortcomings so one's repertoire of sexual interests and breadth of exposure to sexual activities and anatomy can be more adventurous. This idea is supported by research suggesting that from a list of 11 possible sexual activities male respondents place sex involving two males and one female as their 11th favoured behaviour (Husain & Qureshi, 2016), yet analysis of pornography accessed over the Internet has shown that men preferentially view pornography depicting multiple men and one woman over multiple women and a single man (Pound, 2002). Thus, it is plausible that our real-life sexual lives and our fantasy sexual lives linked to pornography may overlap but are not the same.

Upskirting

KS reported that as part of accessing voyeuristic pornography he had started to watch online videos of filming up the skirts and dresses of unsuspecting females. He then experimented with making his own videos. His initial attempts failed but he persevered until he succeeded, suggesting a powerful drive to obtain these images. Interestingly he reported that part of his motivation was to overcome the practicalities of obtaining these pictures and videos, in addition to the sexual interest.

He placed a mobile phone in an adapted holdall and would walk around a large English city pursuing females that he described as attractive and who were wearing skirts or dresses in order to obtain "the perfect shot". Initially his tactics were high risk to himself in that his potential victims often noticed him walking close behind them and would respond negatively to that, although they were unaware that he was attempting to photograph or film under their clothes. A strategy to overcome this need for proximity was to try filming and taking pictures when travelling behind women on escalators. Later his strategy developed further, he would enter department stores with his holdall, and leave it in an aisle between racks of clothes, whilst pretending to browse. His goal was that women would step over the holdall and whilst doing so would expose themselves to his filming without him needing to be nearby and potentially raising suspicions, but still being able to monitor if he might have captured any film or if he needed to reclaim the holdall if it was reported as having been abandoned. He reported that whilst he was engaged in any of his upskirting activity, he was not sexually aroused. KS appreciated that this activity and planning could be construed as "dodgy" but managed any kind of internal conflict by holding on to the thought that he was actually there to buy his mother a gift. So he was relying to some extent on having a plausible narrative that allowed him to overcome internal barriers to offending and potentially to have an explanation should he be questioned as to why he was browsing in the women's clothes section of a shop. So there is some evidence of a conflict between actively pursuing filming opportunities and explaining it to himself as it being opportunistic whilst in a "risky" environment for non-offending reasons.

This shift in tactic suggests a degree of planning and an element of forensic awareness rather than his behaviour being opportunistic or impulsive. He was able to acknowledge that his motivation was ultimately sexual. At the time of the filming, KS' view was that he was focussing on the technical and practical challenges of trying to get footage and was not aroused, but he would watch the material at home and masturbate. His reflection on his upskirting behaviour was that he was attempting to achieve the perfect picture of a woman, something that he was unable to describe. Indeed, he was unable to provide details of preferences such as if the victim was wearing underwear (and if so any preference for colour or type, although he did state, "the sexier the better" but without being able to describe examples of "sexy" underwear), the position of her legs, if she had tights, or leggings, or stockings. This is interesting as without a template of perfection there is no achievable goal and thus there is always a reason to continue taking more pictures and more film because perfection has not been reached; this could be construed as a strategy to give oneself permission to continue to act in ways that one knows is inappropriate. The second component of his understanding of his behaviour was that there was the secrecy of both what the woman was wearing (and that most men would have no knowledge of this) and the secrecy that she would not know that he had managed to gain access to this information. This made him feel powerful and competent. Finally, KS was keen to have new material rather than relying on a small collection that he could view repeatedly, which would have been a safer strategy (but perhaps would have removed the implied closeness to people he could experience by taking pictures, the renewal of power dynamics, and having a greater wealth of "secrets") and it provided him with novel material to use for masturbatory fantasies. KS stated that he did not imagine that any of the women would find his behaviour attractive if they caught him or that it might lead to any form of relationship or sexual behaviour between him and his victims.

KS reported that he always kept the necessary materials with him when he went out. He identified that he had bought the holdall and adapted it in response to watching "YouTube" videos. At that time he was motivated by questions such as "how do they get away with it" and thus setting himself a challenge. When questioned further about this, KS had not considered the possibility that many videos could be staged; thus, there was no risk and no challenge to the film-makers and that the victims of these portrayals would not identify themselves as victims of an offence, rather they may have been paid. This naivety in respect of pornography may be an important consideration when we remember KS' concerns about his own sexual knowledge and skills. If he believed that all pornography is real, that there is no staging or acting involved, he might reasonably assume that real people have the kinds of sex lives portrayed in pornography, that people are as competent and confident as they are portrayed, and that the sex is always enormously successful for everyone involved. For someone who believes that they are unskilled and without knowledge the use of pornography may be both sexually arousing yet negatively impacting on self-confidence. A Swedish study of young men (14–20 years) indicated that pornography can have a negative influence; the young men expressed concerns about their ability to perform as well and for the same duration as the men depicted in the films (Löfgren-Mårtenson & Månsson, 2010).

KS knew what he was doing was risky and that there would be consequences if caught, but his reported excitement of both the process and the resultant videos (his own and other people's) was, he stated, more important at that time. However, this awareness and concern for negative consequences were clearly apparent by his reaction when in treatment he mentioned that he thought he had missed an appointment to sign the sex offender register, which resulted in a degree of stress and KS considering what the implications for him might be, what he might lose. Evidently, in some circumstances he was able to appreciate the negative impact of his own behaviour.

KS uploaded films and images onto his computer to watch at a later date, the files being named and categorised. The extent to which an individual categorises their collections is considered to be important in understanding the seriousness of the offending in people who offend against children (Taylor & Quayle, 2003) and it is reasonable that this holds for other kinds of sexual offending. When KS was caught, he was found to be in possession of approximately 105 videos, which he describes as "the best" ones. From KS' perspective, this was based on a combination of successfully showing the victim's underwear and there being some closeness to his sense of an "ideal". KS was unable to clearly describe this ideal, but had a sense that there was such a thing and once it was captured he would stop. Of course, having an ideal that is not specified gives one the opportunity to never be satisfied and to continue with one's behaviour to achieve a goal. Which is probably unattainable. Good videos were ones of women that he found attractive and that had prolonged film of their underwear, and kind of underwear were important too; "the sexier the better". KS was not able to give an account of what fit the criteria of "sexy" underwear nor what it was that made the women attractive or otherwise. Importantly, in the latter case, given the way that he obtained his pictures and videos the majority would not have contained images of the women's faces and when the films were taken from a shop floor, they were unlikely to contain images of the women's bodies. As such, one might question whether KS was considering "attractive" in the same way that is typical and indeed it may be that this was a strategy to minimise his offending, i.e. "I am not filming all women, only attractive women" which perhaps helps to manage his self-image and provide a rationale for his behaviour, along with suggesting to others that there was a selection process, rather than this being an uninhibited, uncontrolled process, that might imply a greater level of risk.

The videos and pictures were used by KS as fantasy material. He had no videos of women without underwear so was unable to comment on whether this would have been a preference for him and might be more sexually alluring for him. A 2016 YouGov poll (YouGov, 2016) suggests that 3% of women in the UK do not wear any kind of underwear so there was a chance that KS might have had pictures or video of women without underwear but chose to delete them. With regard to the fantasies, KS reported that they are fulfilling because they allow for the use of imagination and determining the outcome of the fantasy, and often this is better than the reality of sex. In relation to this, KS said that the fantasy element of the behaviour is "exactly the same as a first date" but whereas 1st dates are awkward for him; he knows exactly what to do in his fantasies and can determine how the interaction progresses.

KS reported that although he was able to masturbate to both fantasies of *urolagnia* and pornography and upskirting images, the former feels "dirtier" and as such feels more exciting and fulfilling.

Throughout the assessment, KS portrayed himself as having two distinct interests but further investigation into his fantasies demonstrated that there were occasions when the two would be brought together. He discussed ongoing fantasies that were active during the period of the assessment where there were elements of both i.e. seeing a woman in a business suit on the street, walking behind her for perhaps 10s, imagining her hitching up her skirt and urinating. KS considered that this was an unusual fantasy as in his other *urolagnia* fantasies the woman was always imagined in close proximity to the toilet. He also reported that he found these fantasies more difficult to manage, possibly because they did contain features from both of his preferred areas of sexual interest and because he found them highly arousing.

Triggers

KS was able to provide examples of factors that he perceived as triggers that would make him more likely to offend. These triggers were specific to *urolagnia*. The triggers that KS identified were as follows:

Inadvertently having to use a shared toilet immediately after a woman had used it and then unsuccessfully managing thoughts about how that woman might have behaved in the toilet.
Use of cannabis and or alcohol, which reduced his ability to censor his thoughts.
Becoming sexually aroused to thoughts.
Feelings of jealousy about his lack of a relationship (seeing males speaking with women) and concerns that he cannot develop one.
Social isolation, which he manages by drugs, alcohol, and the use of pornography.

An OaSys chart from 2014 identified accommodation, employment, relationships, lifestyle, thinking and behaviour, and attitudes as issues that needed to be addressed to reduce the likelihood of recidivism. Interestingly, neither drug nor alcohol misuse was identified. This may be because to probation he appears to have indicated that he never used drugs and only drank socially.

At the time of the assessment, KS really only had two strategies in place if he started to notice that he was having offence-related thoughts. One was to use aversive thoughts, such as negative thoughts of being caught. The second was to promote thought-stopping through the use of an elastic band on his wrist in response to a particular stimulus; he provided an example where he used this to give himself a sharp pain before thoughts developed in response to seeing a woman in tights. This strategy came from NSORG as they thought, in KS' recollection, that his thinking appeared obsessive. Although KS reported that at times both of these strategies would work they were less effective if he was in a low mood or had been drinking because at these times, in his opinion, by the time he thought about using a strategy he was already engaged in the thinking and the fantasy.

Current Circumstances

KS considers that he is "bone idle" and possibly always has been, perhaps because he has always been taken care of throughout his life. Also in part he considers himself to have a lack of desire to do new things because his view is he is not confident and is not socially competent. This has resulted in a focus on others' views of him—partly due to fears of being identified as an offender as a partial picture and his name was published in the local press—and this prevents him getting involved in things that interest him and to reach his goals. Despite being well educated and a bright individual, he does agency work, mostly in factories, working on the production line, although he has recently moved to a different part of the factory working in the stores. He lives alone in a rented flat and rarely ventures out. An element of this is financial but having lost touch with most of his university friends on account of taking an extra year to finish his degree and due to his offending, he has few social opportunities. His most frequent social outing is to watch football games, either at the ground for home games or in a pub on television for away games, but he is not friends with the people that he will be with in either setting. At the time of assessment, he would meet one male friend for drinks perhaps once every two to three months. He lives in the city where he went to university, which is quite some distance from his original home, where his few relatives live.

Psychometrics

In addition to the clinical assessment, KS responded to a number of psychometric tests:

The Personality Assessment Inventory (PAI)
The Clinical Outcomes in Routine Evaluation (CORE)
The Trauma Symptom Inventory (TSI)
The State-Trait Anger Inventory (Version 2) (STAXI-2)
The Inventory of Altered Self-Capacities (IASC)

The PAI (Morey, 2007) is a self-report measure investigating the aspects of personality and psychopathology, which is often used in forensic settings and has support for its usefulness (see, e.g., Wang et al., 1998). Scores from the PAI suggested a number of personality features that were of interest. KS appeared to downplay negative aspects of himself, including his use of drugs and alcohol. Additionally he appeared to identify the problems with sensation-seeking behaviour, poor interpersonal rapport, feelings of helplessness, and impulsivity. There were no indications of clinical psychopathology. The overview of the PAI scores suggested that he was best characterised as withdrawn and introverted, with a passive interaction style, describing himself as meek and unassertive. However, his responses suggested a positive attitude towards the possibility of change, the value of therapy, and the importance of personal responsibility.

The CORE (Evans et al., 2009) assesses general well-being and social functioning, along with risk to self and others. All of KS' responses were within the range expected for a non-clinical sample of males.

The TSI (Briere, 1995) is a self-report measure of trauma-related symptoms evaluating chronic and acute symptoms, including the effects of sexual assault, early experiences of child abuse, and traumatic loss. KS' scores were within the typical range and he did not endorse any critical items.

The STAXI-2 (Spielberger, 1999) provides a concise measure of the experience and expression of anger. The only scale where KS scored above the clinical threshold was the scale "Anger Expression In (AXI)", a measure of how often angry feelings are felt but suppressed rather than expressed either verbally or physically. This suggests that KS has a tendency to not show his anger, despite feeling it. However, studies have suggested that the STAXI-2 may be susceptible to social desirability response bias (where individuals claim positive attributes rather than deny negative attributes), although the data to data show that where social desirability is influencing clients' responses it is associated with lower reported anger expression (McEwan, Davis, MacKenzie, & Mullen, 2009).

The IASC (Briere & Runtz, 2002) is a self-report measure of an individual's sense of identity, their capacity to tolerate strong emotions without dissociation or coping through substance abuse, and form relationships without having fears of abandonment or engaging in activities that intentionally threaten those relationships, including the client–therapist relationship. These factors have been identified as potentially prone to traumatic events. None of KS' scores suggested problems in any of these areas.

References

Abouesh, A., & Clayton, A. (1999). Compulsive voyeurism and exhibitionism: A clinical response to paroxetine. *Archives of Sexual Behavior, 28*(1), 23–30.

Bogaert, A. F. (2001). Handedness, criminality, and sexual offending. *Neuropsychologia, 39*, 465–469.

Briere, J. (1995). *The trauma symptom inventory professional manual.* Odessa, FL: Psychological Assessment Resources.

Briere, J., & Runtz, M. (2002). The inventory of altered self-capacities (IASC): A standardized measure of identity, affect regulation, and relationship disturbance. *Assessment, 9*(3), 230–239.

Evans, C., Mellor-Clark, J., Margison, F., Barkham, M., Audin, K., Connell, J., & McGrath, G. (2009). CORE: Clinical outcomes in routine evaluation. *Journal of Mental Health, 9*(3), 247–255.

Gaupp, L. A., Stern, R. M., & Ratliff, R. G. (1971). The use of aversion-relief procedures in the treatment of a case of voyeurism. *Behavior Therapy, 2,* 585–588.

Husain, W., & Qureshi, Z. (2016). Preferences in marital sexual practices and the role of pornography. *Sexologies, 25,* 35–41.

Jackson, B. T. (1969). A case study of voyeurism treated by counterconditioning. *Behavioral Research & Therapy, 7,* 133–134.

Lavin, M. (2008). Voyeurism: Psychopathology and theory. In D. Richard Laws & W. T. O'Donohue (Eds.), *Sexual deviance: Theory, assessment, and treatment* (pp. 305–319). New York, NY: The Guilford Press.

Löfgren-Mårtenson, L., & Månsson, S. (2010). Lust, love, and life: A qualitative study of Swedish adolescents' perceptions and experiences with pornography. *Journal of Sex Research, 47,* 568–579.

McEwan, T. E., Davis, M. R., MacKenzie, R., & Mullen, P. E. (2009). The effects of social desirability response bias on STAXI-2 profiles in a clinical forensic sample. *British Journal of Clinical Psychology, 48,* 431–436.

Morey, L. C. (2007). *The personality assessment inventory professional manual.* Lutz, FL: Psychological Assessment Resources.

Nelson, A. (1977). A case of voyeurism (scoptophilia). *The Journal of Orgonomy, 11*(1), 57–61.

Pound, N. (2002). Male interest in visual cues of sperm competition risk. *Evolution and Human Behavior, 23*(6), 443–466.

Spielberger, C. (1999). *STAXI-2 state-trait anger expression inventory-2: Professional manual.* Odessa, FL: Psychological Assessment Resources.

Talbot, T. J., & Langdon, P. E. (2006). A revised sexual knowledge assessment tool for people with intellectual disabilities: Is sexual knowledge related to sexual offending behaviour? *Journal of Intellectual Disability Research, 50*(7), 523–531.

Taylor, M., & Quayle, E. (2003). *Child pornography: An Internet crime.* Hove: Brunner-Routledge.

Wang, E. W., Rogers, R., Giles, C. L., Diamond, P. M., Herrington-Wang, L. E., & Taylor, E. R. (1998). A pilot study of the personality assessment inventory (PAI) in corrections: Assessment of malingering, suicide risk, and aggression in male inmates. *Behavioral Sciences & the Law, 15*(4), 469–482.

YouGov (2016). *The last days of the Y Front.* https://yougov.co.uk/news/2016/08/12/exposed-britains-underwear-preferences-unveiled/.

CHAPTER 7

Clinical Analysis and Formulation

Abstract Based on the information presented in Chapter 6, this chapter presents the analysis and formulation, using the 5Ps model of formulation, laying out the hypothesis for the development and maintenance of KS' offending behaviour, along with identifying the trigger for increasing risk, and the protective factors that have worked to manage his offending.

Keywords *Urolagnia* · Offence paralleling behaviour · Formulation

The process of developing a psychological understanding of someone, which is really a series of hypotheses (Eells, 2007) attempting to show how behaviour may have developed, how it may be maintained, and how it might be changed, is referred to as formulation. It should be regarded as a series of hypotheses, or what Harper and Moss (2003) refer to as perspectives, because even if change occurs, based on the treatment suggested by the formulation, there is not incontrovertible evidence that guarantees that the formulation is correct. A formulation should also be understood as an iterative process; with more information, a formulation may change in important ways, and it is a collaborative process. As Persons (1989) has noted, a formulation should be sensitive to the client's report of the situation and their understanding of it. We are attempting to develop a narrative that examines the underlying

S. Duff, *Voyeurism*, https://doi.org/10.1007/978-3-319-97160-5_7

psychology of the presenting issue and suggest hypotheses for helping to make change. The skill of formulation has been identified as central to clinical psychologists (Kinderman, 2001), and the same view should be held for all applied psychologists. When working with the risk of reoffending, the value of a formulation is that it can provide an explicit description of the clinician's thinking, allowing for critique and shared understanding, along with helping to develop management plans that are based on the evidence that the formulation provides (see Margison & Brown, 2007, for advantages of formulation). Harper and Moss (2003) have suggested that there is no one correct approach to formulation and that a formulation is a map rather than the territory.

There are a variety of models for formulation, varying "in the degree to which they emphasise a collaborative process between clinicians and clients" (MacDonald & Mikes-Liu, 2009, p. 270) and given KS' identified concerns about the unusualness of his behaviour, his social awkwardness, yet being bright, articulate, and reflective, the decision was made to use a model that allows for a high degree of collaboration. Additionally, given my own particular biases in thinking about human behaviour, the formulation needed to reflect a biopsychosocial approach to understanding KS. To this end the Five Ps model (Kuyken, Padesky, & Dudley, 2008) of formulation was used. The benefits of the 5Ps model is that it is easily communicated to clients, the categories can help with the analysis and the focus of the material under consideration, and it provides a degree of motivation and encouragement by including protective factors within the categories. Within forensic work, it is widely used and allows for a degree of flexibility by, for example, allowing for the inclusion of coping strategies within it. The 5Ps are as follows:

Presenting issues—the current problems the person faces in terms of difficult behaviours, emotions, and thoughts. By identifying what are considered to be the issues, and the impact they are having, it is possible to determine short-, medium-, and long-term goals.

Predisposing factors—the likely origins and development of the problems. These may be individual, biological, or contextual factors and it is important to consider both the quantity of these events and the quality of the events. For a given individual having experienced a single traumatic event may have significant consequences similar to experiencing many traumatic events, so the meaning of these events to the individual are important to evaluate.

Precipitating factors—these are the triggers which cause the behaviour or make it more likely to happen and these can be external (e.g. time or place) or internal (thoughts and feelings). It is possible that there are complex series of events which are precipitating factors and it is important to understand the interconnections between various factors. For example, drinking alcohol may link to rumination, rumination may lead to thoughts of lack of intimacy, which in turn may result in sexual frustration, culminating in antisocial decisions to seek sexual stimuli. However, alcohol may not always be the starting point of this process.

Perpetuating factors—these are the factors that maintain the presenting issues. For example, sexual satisfaction may perpetuate voyeurism, as might the desire to have a complete collection of images perpetuate downloading of images of child abuse.

Protective factors—these identify the individual's strengths including personal and social resources that have been useful in preventing the presenting issues from occurring or that help to stop the behaviour once it has begun, or prevent the behaviour from escalating.

To read more about the specifics of this approach see, for example, Delle-Vergini and Day (2016), and Kuyken et al. (2008).

As KS was assessed and treated over an extended period of time, and formulations evolve over time, it is not possible to provide a single formulation that adequately encapsulates that entire period. The formulation presented below is based on the starting point for the intervention, including the data from the psychometrics that were given to KS at the start of the assessment, and it is what drove the intervention. One important decision that was made prior to the formulation that is set out below is that although the two forms of offending are quite different in how they were carried out, they share the underlying theme of voyeurism and appear to be precipitated and perpetuated by the same issues. For these reasons, they are considered here to be expressions of the same psychology, just two different strategies to achieve the same goal (see Table 7.1).

The formulation suggests that although KS' first awareness of females using the toilet was not experienced as sexual or interesting (when he would see his mother), he became more curious once it took on the aspect of being something secret (women would do it away from other people) and something that different women might do in different ways. This curiosity increased as he entered puberty and began to gain an understanding of the differences between males and females and

Table 7.1 5Ps collaborative formulation for KS

5Ps formulation of KS	
Presenting issues	Voyeurism
	Urolagnia
	Upskirting
Predisposing factors	Early experience of seeing females use the toilet
	Developing early interest that became sexualised
	Secret and private, knowledge
	Socially inhibited
	Lack of sexual knowledge
Precipitating factors	Sexually demeaned
	Anger → control and dominance
	Alcohol
	Drug use
	Social isolation
	Boredom
	Feeling low ("life is shit", "I don't have the life I could have had")
	Not being in a relationship/having sex
	Jealousy of others having relationships
	Sexual fantasies
	Pornography
	Hypervigilant
	Using shared toilets
	Finances
Perpetuating factors	Sexual stimulation from pictures and videos
	Secrecy
	Feelings of competence and dominance
	Desire for perfect picture and perfect pose
	Use of pornography
	Challenge
	I will never be good enough for sex—lack of knowledge (no sex for 20 years)
	I cannot change
	Seeking sexual knowledge
	Socially inhibited/fear of recognition
Protective factors	Desire to change/seeking help
	Fear of consequences of voyeurism
	No evidence of escalation or other paraphilias
	Some evidence of management strategies
	Does not offend whilst in relationships
	Well educated
	Employed

through becoming sexually interested in females. The hypothesis is that at this stage his interest in females using the toilet was non-sexual curiosity, and may well have been minimised from his experience of his mother not choosing to use the toilet in private. So there is no pathologising of the mother in this account or the sexualising of her using the toilet. As he was socially inhibited and had limited sexual knowledge, and no sexual experience in his youth, attempts to see females in the toilet was a method to gain some knowledge and to have some sense of competence, along with satisfying his curiosity.

Although he knew nothing directly of sex, it allowed KS to join in when other boys at school spoke of sex, working to reduce his feelings of isolation. As these were his early experiences of any sexual kind, they are likely to have been a part of his early sexual fantasies, possibly continuing into adulthood. The crucial factor for KS was when his last partner was very critical of him sexually; up to that point he believed that his sexual relationships were typical and he had not received any negative feedback regarding his sexual skills or knowledge. Having been sexually demeaned, KS effectively withdrew from sexual encounters with women. At the start this was because he doubted himself but as time passed, and he remained without sexual experience, this was compounded by a concern that he had learned nothing new, that his sexual knowledge and skills would not have evolved and so any new partner would identify this and would reject him and possibly criticise him again. Now being afraid of further criticism, along with his underlying social anxiety, KS felt unable to attempt to develop relationships with women, but still was sexually interested in women and was interested in having a partner. KS was already using pornography and this is likely to be the sole mechanism through which he achieved any form of sexual outlet. The hypothesis is that this is where the voyeurism became a coping mechanism. He felt unable to engage with women because of his anxiety, he had developed a fear of relationships due to criticism and the ensuing concerns regarding his sexual abilities, and was motivated by pornographic depictions of women, including those portraying explicit examples of voyeuristic behaviour. The two central elements that resulted in voyeurism being acted out are that voyeurism allowed KS a degree of intimacy that pornography would not allow, yet it was safe as it did not require that he have any social or sexual contact with women, and that it gave him a method to regain the self-esteem, through power, dominance, and secrecy, that he had lost both through being sexually demeaned and because of his social inhibition. This is also acted out through his hiring of prostitutes to enact *urolagnic* scenes for him, without involving himself with them physically or taking advantage of the freedom he had in this context. He could have viewed them other than from the side, he could have asked that they directly sexually stimulate him, or that he could stimulate them or have intercourse, but on no occasion did he do so. He was however in a position of authority, being able to dictate the terms of the interaction and their behaviour. Interestingly, he did not attempt to photograph the prostitutes nor did he masturbate whilst they were with him. He is unable to provide an explanation for these features but it is plausible that there was little skill involved and as such photographing them would have been entirely sexual (undermining his defence that he was not driven solely by sexual motives, see below) and if he were to masturbate with them in the room, his view could have been that they might have noticed he was naive and unskilled in masturbation.

Once established as a pattern of behaviour to satisfy his two goals, KS found ways to justify the risks he was taking and the continuation of behaviour that he knew was wrong. He established the idea that rather than being sexually driven, there was an element of technical proficiency and skill involved and that he had a goal in achieving sight or record of the perfect image. Both act to minimise what we might consider the "perversity" of his actions and the "infiniteness" of them. It can be construed as art, or perhaps glamour photography, that will conclude when perfection is achieved.

KS' behaviour was more likely to occur in situations when he would ruminate on his circumstances and fears, such as when drinking, using drugs, or experiencing low mood through feeling isolated or jealous. This suggests he would fit well with the third category of voyeur as described by Kaplan and Krueger (1997), where the voyeurism predominantly seems to be triggered by "stress". His low mood was frequently precipitated by comparing his life with the lives of his university contemporaries who he assumed, based on their social media profiles, that they had money and positive relationships. His jealousy was precipitated by this social comparison and when he saw couples in bars and pubs; both the fact that other men had relationships and what he saw as the ease with which men in bars were able to approach women and talk to them. Often his low mood would lead him to use alcohol and drugs as coping mechanisms, which would disinhibit him and result in greater use of pornography. On occasions, this did lead directly to him going to pubs and clubs where he would attempt access to women's toilets. The *urolagnia* appears to be more directly mood-dependent whereas the upskirting appears to be more directly driven by wanting more material for fantasy and to achieve the "perfect" picture. Both provided sexual material, both were gained through stealth and secrecy, and gave KS the sense that he knew things that others didn't know, and that his victims also did not know that he had seen or filmed them. Unfortunately, the voyeurism, although providing a short-term fix for his needs, did not provide a longer-term fix. It did not challenge his sense of poor knowledge and skills, it did not provide social contact, and he was never able to achieve the perfect picture. The fact that there was no change in the areas that KS most wanted change contributed to his sense that he couldn't change—both in not being able to develop sexual skills (and through that challenge his sense that he was a sexual failure) and have a relationship and in not being able to change his inappropriate interests and behaviours.

The precipitating and perpetuating factors perhaps suggest that KS' behaviour was unmanageable, given the underlying goals that he could not meet and the range of factors that were likely to trigger his thoughts and behaviours. However, KS did possess a number of protective factors that had helped him to restrict his voyeurism. As noted earlier, he had a number of strategies that he had developed whilst attending the NSORG programme, such as the use of thought-stopping, although these were not entirely reliable strategies as he had gone on to offend post-treatment. Additionally, he knew that his behaviour was inappropriate and he genuinely appeared to want to change in part due to the potential consequences if he were to keep offending and in part because he believed that voyeurism could not feature in the life that he wanted to live. Having decided that he wanted to change, he then took the next step and he sought assistance. KS' employment was important both because it engaged him, even if only during work hours, but more importantly he was attempting to make a positive change by earning and being in a more socially demanding situation. The fact that the money provided finances to access alcohol and drugs and that he did not develop a strong social network was a negative outcome from a positive intention.

During the entire time of his offending, once it had established itself, there was no evidence of escalation and no thoughts or fantasies involving escalation to contact offences or even publishing his own video material online. Finally, the fact that whilst in relationships he did not engage in any form of voyeurism, nor did he demonstrate what might be termed here offence paralleling behaviour (Daffern et al., 2007) suggests that KS' needs were quite specific. Offence paralleling behaviour (OPB) has been defined as follows: "Any form of offence related behavioural (or fantasized behaviour) pattern that emerges at any point before or after an offence. It does not have to result in an offence; it simply needs to resemble, in some significant respect, the sequence of behaviours leading up to the offence" (Jones, 2004, p. 38). Outside of relationships, clearly he did engage in OPB through fantasies and through the hiring of prostitutes to enact voyeuristic scenes.

References

Daffern, M., Jones, L., Howells, K., Shine, J., Mikton, C., & Tunbridge, V. (2007). Refining the definition of offence paralleling behaviour. *Criminal Behaviour and Mental Health, 17,* 265–273.

Delle-Vergini, V., & Day, A. (2016). Case formulation in forensic practice: Challenges and opportunities. *Journal of Forensic Practice, 18*(3), 240–250.

Eells, T. D. (2007). History and current status of psychotherapy case formulation. In T. D. Eells (Ed.), *Handbook of psychotherapy case formulation* (2nd ed., pp. 3–32). New York: Guilford Press.

Harper, D., & Moss, D. (2003). A different kind of chemistry? Reformulating 'formulation'. *Clinical Psychology, 25,* 6–10.

Jones, L. F. (2004). Offence paralleling behaviour (OPB) as a framework for assessment and interventions with offenders. In A. Needs & G. Towl (Eds.), *Applying psychology to forensic practice.* Oxford: Blackwell and British psychological Society.

Kaplan, M., & Krueger, R. (1997). Voyeurism: Psychopathology and theory. In D. R. Laws & W. O'Donohue (Eds.), *Sexual deviance: Theory, assessment, and treatment* (pp. 297–310). New York, NY: Guilford Press.

Kinderman, P. (2001). The future of clinical psychology training. *Clinical Psychology, 8,* 6–10.

Kuyken, W., Padesky, C. A., & Dudley, R. (2008). The science and practice of case conceptualization. *Behavioural and Cognitive Psychotherapy, 36,* 757–768.

MacDonald, C., & Mikes-Liu, K. (2009). Is there a place for biopsychosocial formulation in a systemic practice? *The Australian and New Zealand Journal of Family Therapy, 30*(4), 269–283.

Margison, F., & Brown, P. (2007). Assessment in psychotherapy. In J. Naismith & S. Grant (Eds.), *Seminars in the psychotherapies* (pp. 1–27). London: RCPsych Publications.

Persons, J. B. (1989). *Cognitive therapy in practice: A case formulation approach.* New York, NY: Norton.

CHAPTER 8

Intervention

Abstract This chapter presents the intervention that was carried out in collaboration with KS, built on the formulation.

Keywords ICASA · Eye movement desensitisation and reprocessing CBT · Covert desensitisation · Victim apology · Perfect voyeurism

The formulation suggested a number of approaches to support KS, a number of which were not feasible in this setting, but are important to mention as they are considered in some areas to be valid interventions. In particular, one could consider the employment of a sex surrogate, known as sexual surrogate partner therapy, which is offered by, amongst other providers, by ICASA (Intimacy Consciousness and Self Awareness) in the UK. Here, the idea is that people with sexual problems can receive intervention that involves engaging in sexual contact with a therapist to overcome, for example, performance anxiety. Their view is stated as "While fear of intimacy may result from background factors and early life conditioning, the solution and a permanent lifelong recovery does not necessarily come from an exhaustive analysis of the causes. Instead, what has been shown to be most effective is a current, direct experience of the healing power of intimacy in the present" (http://www.icasa.co.uk/icasa-self-development-programmes). It is possible that through such an approach, KS would receive informed feedback about his sexual knowledge and skills in a supportive environment and could also

S. Duff, *Voyeurism*, https://doi.org/10.1007/978-3-319-97160-5_8

develop new skills if that was thought necessary. As this appears to be an important basis for KS' behaviour, this might be an effective intervention. However, this is not a service that we are able to refer to. It would be fascinating to discover how many people do access this kind of intervention for paraphilias, as opposed to sexual difficulties such as premature ejaculation, and the impact, if any, that it has.

Another possibility, that was offered to KS but he declined, is eye movement desensitisation and reprocessing (EMDR, Shapiro, 1989) with a view of helping KS manage the trauma of having been criticised by his previous partner. EMDR is recognised for the treatment of traumatic memories and based on KS' description of, and his reactions to, the event of having been sexually demeaned by his last partner, that memory could respond to EMDR. The principle behind EMDR is that trauma interferes with the formation of memory, which in turn can result in unhelpful behaviours and responses. By "reprocessing" the memory, these memories can be appropriately stored and become functional. Our service does offer EMDR and it is regularly used with individuals who have sexually abused and been sexually abused, having been shown to be effective in a variety of cases that involve sexual behaviour as the trauma or as the resulting behaviour (e.g. Cox & Howard, 2007; Parnell, 1999; Wernik, 1993). Importantly, although an accepted intervention, some evidence suggests that it is not effective in all situations and indeed, that the eye-movement part of the therapy is unnecessary (Davidson & Parker, 2001).

From previous case studies, a behavioural approach could have been tried, on the basis that it would appear that an element of KS' behaviour is having learned the benefits of this form of sexual behaviour. It is possible that pairing these behaviours with negative outcomes, such as electric shock, shame, or noxious odours, could result in them losing any value for KS. We don't use such techniques but another concern is that in many of the cases where this approach is described the alternative behaviour is to use pornography. KS already used a range of pornography for sexual purposes, and this doesn't deal with other important areas highlighted in the formulation, such as social anxiety and negative self-belief regarding sexual competence. Clearly one could apply a range of techniques in addition to aversive conditioning, but we do not do this. It would be interesting to know if anyone does regularly rely on aversive techniques to try to change behaviour.

The following provides a description of what was done. For the purposes of brevity, this will not be presented session-by-session, but by theme and approach, with appropriate referencing for the areas that may be less familiar. Overall, it was a CBT approach, making the most of KS' good intellectual reflective abilities. It is also important to note that not every element was successful, or successful in the context of our service, and those occasions will be highlighted, with some possible explanations for their ineffectiveness.

Stage 1—Making KS Safe

The first stage was to develop short duration, powerful approaches to prevent KS from reoffending, before tackling the underlying issues that resulted in voyeurism. The rationale for this was in part practical; if KS were to reoffend, he would likely receive a custodial sentence and although there are programmes for sexual offenders within the prison service, they tend to be more positioned towards offences against children and sexual assault against adults. Equally, these programmes do not explicitly deal with the issues that are hypothesised as central to KS' voyeurism. The other reason to make KS safe was to give him a sense that change was possible and that he could start to gain control over his thinking and behaviour. To manage KS' thinking, we revisited the strategies taught to him by NSORG, namely thought-stopping by the use of an elastic band. This was specifically to thoughts of voyeurism or of particular women (either walking near him in skirts or going towards a toilet). To manage negative thoughts that could act as a trigger, we identified a range of areas that he might be able to distract himself to think about more positive things, such as an upcoming gig he was attending, plans he had with friends, along with managing his drinking by only going out with enough money for two drinks. A distraction strategy seemed appropriate as KS was able to provide examples where this had happened naturally. For example, he noted a time when he acknowledges that he had been in a risky situation (for him), where he could have acted, but due to other concerns at the time (getting petrol) he forgot, and then when it came to mind again did not bother to turn around as the immediate idea had passed.

Simple practical methods were also put in place. For example, KS recognised that often when he was out at a bar or restaurant he would, perhaps unconsciously, pick a table, or orientate his chair, so he could see the toilets. He agreed that he would consciously pick places to sit that did not give him a view of the toilets and that did not give him a view of the route to the toilets. If he found himself in a place where that was not possible, he would go elsewhere. KS also agreed that he would try to limit his pornography use to material that did not involve upskirting or any form of explicit voyeurism. Finally, he agreed to keep a diary in order to identify when he had thoughts or fantasies of voyeurism and to try to identify the circumstances when that happened, such as where he was, what he was doing, what he was thinking, and what he was feeling. Over the course of several weeks, KS reported that he was more vigilant about his behaviour and had made a number of practical decisions based on keeping his diary. He started to restrict going to the pub to times when there were football games being shown on television. His view was that he was less likely to notice women and thinking about them using the toilet and less likely to notice men and women talking together as his focus would be on the game. He also reported that when alone at home, when he might normally fill the time with pornography use he had begun to use the time to keep his flat clean, staying on top of dishes, laundry, and shopping. He was also able to distract himself by listening to music and watching non-pornographic videos on the Internet.

Stage 2—Reframing Sex

Refraining from offending was a consistent task for KS but as he was reporting success in finding strategies to deal with some of his triggers and in managing offence-related thoughts and fantasies we agreed to move on to confront what we hypothesised was the primary triggering event for his voyeurism, being sexually demeaned by his last partner (for the sake of writing she will be referred to as Daria). In trying to reframe this, KS was initially only able to accept an explanation where he was at fault, i.e. that he was bad at sex and ignorant of sexual matters, and that Daria and all previous partners must have tolerated his ineptitude and inexperience. By exploring how people might form an opinion of what counts as good sex and good sexual knowledge in a partner we were able to collaborate to generate a number of different possibilities;

Daria may have had sexual partners and had some expectations of what sex would be like.

Daria and KS may have been sexually incompatible in a variety of ways for example, differing interests in sex.

Daria may have had sexual partners who were unusually experienced and experimental and as such she had unusually high expectations.

Daria may have a very specific view of what counts as sex and if sex does not include certain activities, then it is not "good" sex.

Daria may be basing her expectations on what other people have said, what she has read, pornography she has watched, rather than on experience, and have expected that KS could fulfil these expectations despite Daria not telling him what they were.

Daria may have been sexually satisfied in her relationship with KS but at that time wanted to hurt him for some reason.

Daria may have been sexually satisfied in her relationship with KS but at that time wanted to end the relationship.

There are doubtless other possible interpretations but the importance of this process was to confront KS with two possibilities. One was that he cannot know what the reasons were for Daria demeaning him might have been so realistically any explanation he could come up with is as good as any other. The fact that he picked the one explanation that put responsibility entirely on him and implied that he was catastrophically incapable at sex did not make it a valid explanation. Second, it is possible that Daria's comments on his sexual knowledge and skills may have been in comparison with her having unusually high expectations, rather than suggesting he was less skilled and less knowledgeable than the average British male. KS struggled with accepting any of these possible interpretations for a number of reasons. Primarily it was because as unsettling as it was for him, he was used to believing the explanation that put him at fault, but additionally he had no evidence to support any other explanation (i.e. having not had sex since he had no received any compliments nor did he have experience to counter this explanation) and by accepting another explanation he felt he would have to accept that a false belief had contributed to him avoiding sex and relationships for 20 years. The latter was a large barrier for KS as it fed into his concerns that all his peers had done well and that he had achieved nothing, and this would be another contributing factor to the belief that he was a failure through self-defeat (he latterly blamed his laziness and lack of foresight for his poor university degree and hence poor employment prospects). To tackle this issue, we examined evidence for KS' ability to succeed and to change (see below).

Having explored the possibility that there were other explanations we considered if there were ways to find evidence that, at least in part, other explanations might be as likely. KS reported that this was a strategy he had considered in the past. He had considered hiring an escort to directly deal with "the monkey on my back". He did not follow this course of action because he was concerned that he might not be able to rely on the escort to be honest (he felt that if he was paying she would feel obliged to compliment his skills) and he was concerned about the legality, cost, and possible exposure to sexually transmitted diseases. Although he denied, it is reasonable to hypothesise that he was also concerned that an escort might not be positive. KS had not considered that there might be a wealth of educational (not pornographic) material available in libraries and online that he could access, which focus on sexual and relationship education. It is possible that he was aware of this but was concerned that this might provide evidence that he was unknowledgeable. KS was encouraged to find ways to learn more about typical sexual behaviour. Over the time of his work with our service, he did not appear to have taken up this challenge.

KS had an overriding concern that he was a failure and as such we looked at evidence to support and refute this idea. He was very able to provide examples of failure but almost entirely incapable of identifying success. He had recently had a small promotion at work, which he minimised but with some effort could perceive that out of a pool of some 40 people he had been identified as the person to promote. Having accepted this, he was able to identify some possible, positive reasons for why he had been chosen (reliable, hardworking) and with some effort could accept the possibility that these were traits of him now. Thus, he was capable of change (becoming hardworking and reliable) and that of being successful. We also challenged the notion that he was lazy and unmotivated on the basis that he had asked to be referred to our service and had continued to engage with the work, even when it was difficult to schedule around his shift-work. As the work progressed to challenge KS to examine some of his entrenched beliefs about his social competence, he was able to find more evidence of change and motivation, but it was notable that these did not generalise to beliefs about relationships and sex.

Stage 3—Relationships

KS considered that he was socially incompetent (in sessions he was talkative, amusing, engaging) and despite wanting to form relationships felt he was unable to do so. He stated that he is looking for companionship and friendship. The first step was to examine the extent to which he did have relationships of any kind. KS was able to identify a small group of friends that would occasionally meet with, which he considered to be his only relationships. When we looked at his experiences at work KS did acknowledge that there were a number of people that he would talk to on breaks. Not only was he able to conclude that these were relationships and maybe even friendships, but also that these people would actively approach him for conversations, suggesting that they enjoyed his company. KS analysis was that when he was not thinking about interacting with people, it would naturally happen and he didn't think about it, but when he wanted to interact with someone that is when he would become anxious and awkward. By taking one such casual relationship that he had recently formed, we were able to construct a timeline of the initial interactions to identify how the relationship had built up over time and if it was possible to identify strategies and techniques to extract from this, to apply in a more purposeful way. The most basic of these was KS noticed that what had been very utilitarian, work-based dialogues became more general conversations when a non-work topic was introduced after several conversations. We developed that as a strategy, identified a number of work colleagues that KS was already having work-based conversations with, and he committed to finding opportunities to bring new themes into those conversations. For KS these were less "natural" as we had identified who he had to speak with, but he was armed with a method to engage them. He reported that although he only tried this approach once that it had been successful and that he would try it again. Of course, KS was operating within an environment that he knew and with people that he had some knowledge of. The next task was for KS to practise in more challenging environments. We identified an Internet-based social site that gave people opportunities to engage in experiences, such as visiting historic buildings, which only took place if there was a pre-determined number of people attending. KS selected a number of activities that would interest him (in case he felt unable to interact with people, or they were not very encouraging) and he signed up for those meetings. He reported back that he had made the effort to speak with several people and that people had independently engaged with him, again demonstrating to him that he did have the necessary skills to socialise and that people found him interesting company. Although the primary reason was to challenge KS view of himself it was also to provide him with the chance to develop a greater social network and reduce his feelings of social isolation. Although unlikely in the short term (plus the social network was not a dating network), greater exposure to people also increases his chances of developing intimate relationships, which are protective and may allow him to more naturally discover if his concerns about his sexual behaviour are realistic.

The above efforts to improve KS's contacts with others were not specifically targeted at women, but these were considered important elements of KS being able to form relationships. Whereas KS could see that one could change the focus of a conversation through adding in something trivial, making it more social than work-focussed, he reported that if he were thinking about talking to a woman he is unable to think of anything that might work. Some of his previous social interactions show that he is able to negotiate quite complex situations with women, such as getting to know them in social situations, giving them lifts, being a source of support and comfort along with going out to the cinema. By analysing these past situations, KS was able to acknowledge that his behaviour is unlikely to be perceived uncommon or unexpected in these situations; otherwise, they would be infrequent and perhaps stand out as being unsuccessful. As such, his concerns were more about his own worries, analyses, and expectations. As before, we explored examples from his past and at work where he was able to find strategies that worked in low-risk situations and then apply them to either initiating, or changing the focus, of conversations. KS reported that he was able to do this, but was concerned that it was easy to "talk nonsense" but he wouldn't be able to talk about anything or greater importance with a woman. KS identified that the two things he would find most difficult to talk to a woman about would be his offending and his sense of low self-esteem. With his permission, a female colleague, whom he had no previous contact with, came to one of the sessions, and KS engaged her in conversation about both these topics and answered her questions. She then provided feedback about how he had done, how it had made her feel, and her opinions of his abilities. KS was surprised that he was considered to be competent and engaging and the session was remarkably successful in challenging his beliefs about how well he could manage talking about difficult material to a previously unknown woman. Subsequently, he reported that he had felt more confident talking to female colleagues at work and when he attended the social meetings he had joined. He also recalled that at one time he had been asked by a woman to join an amateur theatre group and by his own account he had "got on really well with everyone".

An important element of this work was also to provide KS with the necessary skills to deal with social adversity. He would meet people that would not like him, wouldn't want to speak to him, wouldn't want to be involved with him romantically and as such we considered how one copes with these kinds of negative outcomes. In some ways, KS was an expert because he had the expectation that he would fail socially. Mostly then he had avoided people, but at the times when he didn't or couldn't, he expected a negative outcome, but he stated that he didn't take these personally. He was able to accept that at the very basic level not everyone gets on, and then constructed a list of reasons why in particular circumstances people might not get on. For example, if people at work had recently changed to a night shift they might be less inclined to talk in the first few shifts, or if someone had experienced a negative life event or if they were preoccupied with other tasks. KS' view was that in the circumstances that he could envisage, he would be able to cope with negative social feedback.

Stage 4—Offending

KS had made good progress with addressing a number of the predisposing, precipitating, and perpetuating factors and was reporting that he had fewer offence-supportive thoughts, was using less offence-related pornography, and had experienced no near-miss events. Although this was very positive, all of this work was based on KS' life being positive. So, we had not considered how he would manage if he were to experience some kind of trauma such as a death in the family. For that reason, it was important to directly addressing his offending behaviour. This consisted of a number of stages.

(i) Covert desensitisation—KS acknowledged that the work he had done thus far was founded on the idea that he would successfully be able to distract himself and thought-stop, and moderate his alcohol and drug use. Also that he would find ways to manage the occurrence of low mood. We agreed that all of these strategies were new for him and although he had remained offence free for approximately 6 months this may have been coincidental, more linked to his life currently progressing well rather than the effectiveness and robustness of the intervention. KS wanted to have a greater concern regarding the consequences of his voyeurism; although having fears of prison in the past, this had not proved fool-proof. He thought he was more likely to be scared by having attention brought to his behaviour, where a single victim becomes joined by a group of angry people who are becoming threatening. To this end, we engaged in covert sensitisation in response to two scenarios—KS following a woman in a skirt and KS entering female toilets. In the former situation, KS was asked to generate a detailed image of himself in his home town, noticing a woman in a skirt, and beginning to wonder what kind of underwear she had on, then following her, with the intention of trying to look under her skirt or to try to take a picture. As he approaches behind her, he was directed to imagine her turning around and shouting loudly in his face, demanding to know what he is doing, calling him a pervert, gradually a crowd gathers and they all begin to shout and name-call and jostle him, until eventually he is rescued from the crowd by the police who bundle him into a car. The second scenario required KS to imagine noticing a woman entering the female toilets, him waiting for a few moments before walking in, entering the empty cubicle, and climbing onto the toilet cistern so that he could look over the partition at the woman. As he imagines standing on the cistern and beginning to rise over the partition he was directed to imagine that another woman enters the toilet and sees him, immediately she calls back through the toilet door and a crowd of people come into the toilet, shouting at him, insulting him, and pulling him off the cistern, where he is also confronted by the woman from the other cubicle, who also berates him. As the crowd gets angrier and louder, the police arrive and take him away. KS worked on imagining both of these scenarios over a number of sessions and to practise at home if, for example, he was watching pornography and started to think about images linked to his voyeurism. He reported that he found this effective, even if he was experiencing feelings of loneliness, and that as he practised these routines he would feel gradually more anxious as the imagined scenes progressed. To support KS further, we also focussed on an avoidance strategy, whereby in both cases he noticed the woman, started to follow her (either in the street or towards the toilet) and as he reported starting to feel anxious he was directed to imagine turning away from the woman, no longer following her, and experiencing a great sense of relief, relaxation, and feeling good about himself. KS also practised these scenarios at home.

(ii) Victim Apology—The other part of working on KS' offences was to write a victim apology letter. This is a fairly standard practice when working with sexual offenders (Duff, 2010) and also has been used as a method to identify needs and to examine change after intervention

(Cahalane & Duff, 2018; Cahalane, Duff, & Parker, 2013; Duff, 2011). The strategy was for KS to identify one of his victims and write a letter to her, expressing how he thought that his behaviour might have impacted upon her, so giving some thought to the consequences of his actions. Although KS understood the nature of the task, it was clear from his letter that he had struggled with providing any level of detail as to how a victim might have felt at the time of the offence, how it might have affected them immediately after the offence, and in the longer term. Discussion with KS identified a number of reasons why this exercise may have been useful for him. KS did not have any direct contact with his victims, either at the time of his offences of when convicted. To some extent it was difficult for him to construe them as real people and real victims. Intellectually he understood that he had done wrong and had invaded their privacy, but emotionally he was unable to connect with, for example, a sense of fear, humiliation, or anger that they might have experienced. He genuinely had no idea what impact his behaviour may have had in the long term, despite having a very clear understanding of the possible long-term consequences of others' behaviour, due to the impact of "Daria" on his life. The other possible contributor to this difficulty for KS was his long-term use of pornography. This will have presented voyeurism as harmless, or potentially as eventually leading to the victim and voyeur engaging in sex; thus, he had a general view that voyeurism doesn't really matter to the victim, as they are unlikely to know (which relates back to Doyle's view of perfect voyeurism, Doyle, 2009). As KS did not undertake a letter writing task at the start and end of the intervention, it was not possible to examine if this might have been a method to examine subtle changes in a voyeur, such as victim empathy, or their understanding of their offences.

References

Cahalane, H., & Duff, S. (2018). A qualitative analysis of nonoffending partners' experiences and perceptions following a psychoeducational group intervention. *Journal of Sexual Aggression: An International, Interdisciplinary Forum for Research, Theory and Practice, 24,* 66–79.

Cahalane, H., Duff, S., & Parker, G. (2013). Treatment implications arising from a qualitative analysis of letters written by the nonoffending partners of men who have perpetrated child sexual abuse. *Journal of Child Sexual Abuse, 22*(6), 720–741.

Cox, R. P., & Howard, M. D. (2007). Utilization of EMDR in the treatment of sexual addiction: A case study. *Sexual Addiction and Compulsivity, 14*(1), 1–20.

Davidson, P. R., & Parker, C. H. (2001). Eye movement desensitization and reprocessing (EMDR): A meta-analysis. *Journal of Consulting and Clinical Psychology, 69*(2), 305–316.

Doyle, T. (2009). Privacy and perfect voyeurism. *Ethics and Information Technology, 11*, 181–189.

Duff, S. C. (2010). Exploring criminogenic need through victim apology letters: An interpretative phenomenological analysis. *Journal of Aggression, Conflict and Peace Research, 2*(2), 33–43.

Duff, S. C. (2011). Exploring criminogenic need through victim apology letters II: An IPA analysis of post-treatment accounts of offending against children. *Journal of Aggression, Conflict and Peace Research, 3*(4), 230–242.

Parnell, L. (1999). *EMDR in the treatment of adults abused as children*. New York, NY: Norton.

Shapiro, F. (1989). Efficacy of the eye movement desensitization procedure in the treatment of traumatic memories. *Journal of Traumatic Stress, 2*, 199–223.

Wernik, U. (1993). The role of traumatic component in the etiology of sexual dysfunctions and its treatment with eye movement desensitization procedure. *Journal of Sex Education and Therapy, 19*, 212–222.

CHAPTER 9

Outcomes and Discussion

Abstract This is the discussion of the outcomes of the intervention with KS, which was successful at one level, given that by all accounts he has remained offence free up to the present day. However, it also identifies that there remain a number of vulnerabilities that continue to put KS at risk of reoffending if he does not address them.

Keywords Voyeurism · Psycho-educational approaches Learning-theory · CBT

At a very simplistic level the outcome of working with KS has been successful in that to date he still has not reoffended and as of June 2018 this is still the case. He reports that he does not think of carrying out voyeuristic acts, has not had any near misses, and has completely changed the focus of his pornography use and masturbatory fantasies. Although the pornography, by its nature, still does have a strong voyeuristic element (his preference is for pornography that depicts women masturbating) it does not involve explicit narratives or presentations of voyeuristic strategies and behaviour nor any form or *urolagnia*. He is employed, engages in social groups, but still lives a relatively solitary, isolated life, although he acknowledges that in part this is because he works shifts, which impacts on when he is available to socialise, and that his contemporaries have all got busy lives too. He has not had any form of romantic interaction, not even a date, and has not engaged in any form of sexual

S. Duff, *Voyeurism*, https://doi.org/10.1007/978-3-319-97160-5_9

contact with a woman. This does still cause him a degree of concern, but interestingly now he interprets this as being as a result of his "cowardice" of approaching women rather than because he explicitly expects to be rejected. He is not good at generating his own possibilities for finding opportunities to be around people, nor strategies to engage with people. He has not attempted to educate himself in sexual behaviour. So to some extent the work has been successful, but some of the underlying areas that might further reduce his risk are still extant. From the perspective of risk this is a matter for concern, but perhaps no more than when working with people who are sexually attracted to children. We do not claim that we are changing that sexual attraction, rather giving people the understanding for why acting on that attraction is illegal and damaging, and strategies to avoid and manage risky situations and thoughts, we support them in preventing the attraction from becoming action. We also need to consider the possibility that much of KS' change may be a result of maturation and perhaps his sexual interests have simply changed over time.

Having reached this point KS' concerns have changed and he is reflecting more on having not lived the life that he wished he had. He feels that he has not achieved his full potential and in comparison with his peers he has fallen short. This is both within the spheres of success at work and success within relationships. He has a strategy to deal with what he sees as his shortfalls in work, less so in his relationships, and he sees that as a continuing odyssey that will demand he exposes himself to more social risk and makes the effort to learn more about intimacy and sex.

This is the first, detailed case study of a voyeur and it offers the opportunity to examine, in some depth, how his offending developed and how we might understand the psychology underpinning it. KS has experienced a number of issues that could have led to a number of different interpretations. For example, the fact that from an early age he was exposed to his mother using the toilet might be understood within a psychodynamic framework as being importantly causal. It may have played a part in determining the kinds of coping behaviour KS resorted to when he was triggered to find ways to cope with fear of intimacy but that makes it no more important than, for example, KS' food preferences and certainly less important that the cognition that led him to find the idea of women going to the toilet as curious. This perhaps is the crux of KS' voyeurism, a curiosity that became a part of his pornographic interests, which then was an obvious strategy to gain some level of sexual satisfaction once the typical routes of satisfaction through sexual contact with consenting partners was no longer a "safe" choice. Rather than find a way to challenge Daria's accusations, either intellectually or through further education and experience, he resorted to secret methods, which he could rationalise as challenging (so not entirely aberrant and shameful) and that prevented the chance of further threats to his self-esteem. The effort to do this was more immediately satisfying than the effort and risk of addressing his real concerns. For KS the danger is that if his sexual interests change again or he ceases to care about the consequences of further offending he may again resort to voyeurism.

What does this tell us more generally about voyeurism? As stated at the start of this case study we always have to be cautious about case studies as they cannot extract the specifics of the person. KS is a particular kind of voyeur and reached that point of his behaviour through a particular route, which, hopefully, the formulation provides a helpful map to describe that journey. However, there may be some useful pointers to consider for the assessment of voyeurs.

Firstly is to consider the possibility that rather than voyeurism being the result of some kind of sexual aberration that is due to inherent deviancy, it is a coping mechanism. As such we are provoked to examine what it copes for. Is it to provide access to viewing a particular kind of behaviour, that could indicate a developmental or trauma issue? The reasons for seeking opportunities to see people undressing may be different to seeking opportunities to see people defecating, and it is important to unpick these different kinds of voyeurism and determine if they are underpinned by the same psychology or not. Even if the same psychology is at play we would want to know why in one person it is expressed as viewing someone undressing through a window versus viewing someone using a toilet. The hypothesis for KS' interest in *urolagnia* is that he was seeking knowledge about women, about their behaviour, what makes them different to men and to each other, to give him some form of sexual knowledge and to experience a sense of power-through-secrecy. KS couldn't get this information through direct contact with women and was not prepared to find other ways to learn. Similarly with his *upskirting*, it was a strategy to have a false sense of intimacy, both intellectual and sexual, without the costs of achieving these goals through other means.

If we can identify that coping is a plausible explanation, the next stage is to investigate why voyeurism has been favoured as a coping mechanism and are there other ways that the person could cope. One method could be to entirely rely on pornography as that would keep him from causing harm and upset in the community. This has its own risks, as clinical experience has shown that some people broaden their pornographic palette to start to include more and more extreme kinds of behaviour, which can result in online offending. It also would not tackle the underlying risk issues nor take into consideration an individual's quality of life. To solely rely on pornography, when other prosocial options are available does seem like an impoverished life. In KS' case, he could educate himself, he could practise social skills, he could develop relationships, he could have sex, but these are longer term, potentially risky courses of action. He is stymied by perceiving these routes as risky and, in his own words, being "lazy". He appears to be more interested in finding ways to force change in a top-down manner, rather than bottom-up. This may always leave him vulnerable. Interestingly these are skills that most of us take for granted and many of us have no sense of how we developed these skills. Yet, they are involved in very complex processes, managing the interaction between people, the gradual escalation of intimacy and self-disclosure, and then engaging in behaviour that may be anxiety provoking as we expose ourselves sexually. Perhaps our rudimentary ideas about sexual education need to take into account this complexity and in doing so we may inadvertently provide vulnerable individuals with the knowledge and skills they need to prevent them developing antisocial coping mechanisms.

It would be useful to explore the aspects of a voyeur's self-esteem in a variety of areas, particularly linked to relationships and sex and microscopically analyse that individual's past romantic and sexual experiences. Have they felt sexually demeaned or threatened, do they have concerns about their sexual abilities (whether from experience or hypothetically), their sexual knowledge, their sexual behaviour? Given the ubiquity of pornography, presenting an artificial sense of sex and what people know, do, how effective it is, it is not surprising that vulnerable people will develop a sense of sexual behaviour that may feel far beyond their reach and if it is unobtainable through socially acceptable routes they may find other ways to have some semblance of a sexual life. It is possible that other paraphilia are similar coping mechanisms. The challenge is to find ways to support an individual's self-esteem in ways that are linked to social and sexual contact and this may be difficult with an individual whose self-esteem in those areas is so very fragile.

From the perspective of how KS was treated, having identified a variety of underlying issues these were approached in a variety of ways including CBT, psycho-educational approaches, and learning-theory-driven methods. Many of the previous case studies of voyeurs suggest that there is one underlying problem and one way to tackle it, which is insulting to individuals and to human psychology. Very few of our behaviours have a single, simple cause and theories of behaviour that don't reflect the interaction between experiences, biology, biases, society, the individual's immediate context, and cognition are unlikely to give us the information that we need to support people in changing. It is also important to try not to dismiss particular approaches if one does not believe in them. It would have been possible to ignore KS' early exposure to his mother using the toilet, as KS did, as that might imply a psychodynamic interpretation of his behaviour and had the consequence of interfering with KS' relationship with his mother, which has been and continues to be very positive and supportive. Indeed, KS' mother is one of his strongest sources of social contact. Different approaches suggest different areas of focus, different kinds of information to gather, and by trying to be comprehensive in understanding the people we work with we hope to serve them more effectively and more ethically.

Most importantly, the message from this exercise is that it is clear that we know very little of voyeurs and voyeurism. As it may primarily take place without anyone knowing, we might not have a sense of how common it is and may be of the view that what we don't know doesn't hurt us. However, even if only thinking about the quality of life of voyeurs, the possibility that it may escalate, we need to know more, we need to take it seriously, and we need to find ways to help and understand these individuals.

Glossary

Affordances this theory suggests that not only do we perceive shapes and the relationships between objects (such as A is to the side of B), but also what objects could be used for. Flat surfaces that are raised off the ground and can support weight can have other items put on them, and we class these objects as "tables"

Antiandrogens a class of drugs that prevent the functioning of sex hormones, which can be used in the treatment of sexual offending. They are also used in medical treatment, such as therapy for prostate cancer

Bottom-up a kind of processing of information that is data driven, where the basic constituents of information are gradually linked together to form a more complex representation

Cisgender the description of a person where their personal identity and gender correspond with their sex at birth

Cognitive analytic therapy (CAT) a collaborative therapeutic approach that seeks to work with emotional distress and problems in relationships, recognising the patterns of behaviour and attempting to find ways to change unhelpful patterns that have left the individual stuck in ways of dealing with people

Cognitive behavioural therapy (CBT) a therapeutic approach that seeks to help people manage their problems by addressing how they think and how they behave, by analysing a person's thoughts, physical feelings, emotions, and actions

Coprophilia a sexual interest that involves faeces in some way, for example the sight, smell, touch, or taste

S. Duff, *Voyeurism*, https://doi.org/10.1007/978-3-319-97160-5

Crotch-watching an activity whereby women and men will look at the crotch area of men, particularly with an intention to identify sexual arousal

Exhibitionism where a person voluntarily displays a part of their body not typically made available for public view, in public, or to a non-consenting person. Typically, this includes a man's penis, a woman's breasts, but may include complete nudity

Eye movement desensitisation and reprocessing (EMDR) a psychotherapeutic treatment aimed at managing trauma by reprocessing traumatic memories through bi-lateral stimulation, frequently achieved through moving the eyes back and forth

Frotteurism the act of rubbing a part of oneself, usually the genitals, against another non-consenting individual

Iconophilia a term used to describe a love of images, which can also describe a sexual arousal to images

Innate releasing mechanism (IRM) a proposed cognitive system whereby an automatic behavioural response is triggered when activated by a specific stimulus. For example, ducklings are thought to have an IRM to a moving object, and that explains why they follow their mother. However, this can be triggered by other moving objects, which explains why ducklings will also follow people or other animals if that is what they see at the appropriate developmental stage

Mindfulness a technique that encourages people to bring the focus of their attention to the present moment, rather than fixating on the past or the future. Proponents suggest that it can have a positive impact upon mental health

Northumbria sex offender group programme (NSOGP) a group programme for male sexual offenders, aged 21 and above, who have committed contact and non-contact offences, broadly using a cognitive behavioural (CBT) approach

Occam's razor a principle attributed to the fourteenth-century Franciscan friar and philosopher William of Ockham (1287–1347), which can be expressed as when you have two competing theories that make exactly the same predictions, the simpler one is the better

Offence paralleling behaviour (OPB) Any form of offence-related behavioural (or fantasised behaviour) pattern that emerges at any point before or after an offence. It does not have to result in an offence; it simply needs to resemble, in some significant respect, the sequence of behaviours leading up to the offence.

Pathologise treating something as psychologically abnormal or of concern

Perinatal influences those influences that occur around the time of birth, both before and for a short period afterwards

Postnatal influences those influences that occur after birth, including into childhood, adolescence, and adulthood

Revenge Pornography the sharing of sexually explicit material without the consent of other individuals involved. The material may have been made with the person's consent, or in secret, but it is the sharing that identifies it as revenge pornography

Schema therapy a therapeutic technique that seeks to identify self-defeating patterns of thinking and behaviour (schemas) that developed in childhood and to develop more helpful schema, through a variety of techniques such as visualisation and chair work

Scopophilia a sexual interest in looking at other people's bodies

Top-down a form of processing whereby our beliefs and expectations tend to drive cognition, rather than the actual information in the environment

Troilism the activity whereby two people are having sex and a third person secretly watches. Importantly, for this to be troilism rather than voyeurism, at least one of the two people engaging in sex knows that they are being observed

Zoophilia a sexual interest in non-human animals, also known as bestiality (although experts suggest that zoophilia describes people who form emotional and sexual attachments to animals whereas bestiality describes people who sexually abuse animals)

Bibliography

Abel, G. G., Becker, J. V., Mittelman, M., Cunningham-Rather, J., Rouleau, J. L., & Murphy, W. D. (1987). Self-reported sex crimes of nonincarcerated paraphiliacs. *Journal of Interpersonal Violence, 2*(1), 3–25.

Abel, G. G., & Blanchard, E. B. (1974). The role of fantasy in the treatment of sexual deviation. *Archives of General Psychiatry, 30,* 467–475.

Abel, G. G., Obsorn, C., & Twigg, D. (1993). Sexual assault through the life span: Adult offenders with juvenile histories. In H. E. Barbaree, W. Marshall, & S. M. Hudson (Eds.), *The juvenile sex offender* (pp. 104–117). New York: Guilford Press.

Abouesh, A., & Clayton, A. (1999). Compulsive voyeurism and exhibitionism: A clinical response to paroxetine. *Archives of Sexual Behavior, 28*(1), 23–30.

Ahlers, C. J., Schaefer, G. A., Mundt, I. A., Roll, S., Englert, H., Willich, S. N., et al. (2011). How unusual are the contents of the paraphilias? Paraphilia-associated sexual arousal patterns in a community-based sample of men. *Journal of Sexual Medicine, 8,* 1362–1370.

Allen, C. (1969). *A textbook of psychosexual disorders* (2nd ed.). London: Oxford University Press.

Almeida, O. P., Waterreus, A., Spry, N., Flicker, L., & Martins, R. N. (2004). One year follow-up study of the association between chemical castration, sex hormones, beta-amyloid, memory and depression in men. *Psychoneuroendocrinology, 29*(8), 1071–1081.

American Psychiatric Association. (2000). *Diagnostic and statistical manual of mental disorders* (4th ed., text revision). Washington, DC: Author.

Bandura, A. (1965). Behavior modification through modeling procedures. In L. Krasner, & L. P. Ullman (Eds.), *Research in Behavior Modification.* NY: Holt, Rinehart and Winston.

S. Duff, *Voyeurism*, https://doi.org/10.1007/978-3-319-97160-5

Bandura, A. (1977). *Social learning theory.* NY: Prentice-Hall.

Becker, J. V., & Kaplan, M. S. (1988). The assessment of adolescent sexual offenders. In R. J. Prinz (Ed.), *Advances in behavioural assessment of children and families* (pp. 97–118). Conn: JAI Press Inc.

Bogaert, A. F. (2001). Handedness, criminality, and sexual offending. *Neuropsychologia, 39,* 465–469.

Bond, I. K., & Evans, D. R. (1967). Avoidance therapy: Its use in two cases of underwear fetishism. *Canadian Medical Association Journal, 96*(16), 1160–1162.

Bradford, J. M. W., & Pawlak, A. (1993). Double-blind placebo crossover study of cyproterone acetate in the treatment of the paraphilias. *Archives of Sexual Behavior, 22*(5), 383–402.

Briere, J. (1995). *The trauma symptom inventory professional manual.* Odessa, FL: Psychological Assessment Resources.

Briere, J., & Runtz, M. (2002). The inventory of altered self-capacities (IASC): A standardized measure of identity, affect regulation, and relationship disturbance. *Assessment, 9*(3), 230–239.

Briken, P., Habermann, N., Berner, W., & Hill, A. (2005). The influence of brain abnormalities on psychosocial development, criminal history and paraphilias in sexual murderers. *Journal of Forensic Science, 50,* 1204–1208.

Brown, S. (2005). *Treating sex offenders: An introduction to sex offender treatment programmes.* Cullompton, Devon: Willan Publishing.

Cahalane, H., & Duff, S. (2018). A qualitative analysis of nonoffending partners' experiences and perceptions following a psychoeducational group intervention. *Journal of Sexual Aggression: An International, Interdisciplinary Forum for Research, Theory and Practice, 24,* 66–79.

Cahalane, H., Duff, S., & Parker, G. (2013). Treatment implications arising from a qualitative analysis of letters written by the nonoffending partners of men who have perpetrated child sexual abuse. *Journal of Child Sexual Abuse, 22*(6), 720–741.

Carlin, J. D., & Calder, A. J. (2013). The neural basis of eye gaze processing. *Current Opinion in Neurobiology, 23,* 450–455.

Caron, F., Godin, G., Otis, J., & Lambert, L. D. (2004). Evaluation of a theoretically based AIDS/STD peer education program on postponing sexual intercourse and on condom use among adolescents attending high school. *Health Education Research, 19*(2), 185–197.

Cautela, J. R. (1967). Covert sensitization. *Psychological Reports, 20*(2), 459–468.

Challinor, L. (2015). The perceptions of sex offenders: A comparison of professionals and paraprofessionals in a forensic environment and the general public. *Forensic Update, 117,* 32–36.

Coleman, J. (1964). *Abnormal psychology and modern life* (3rd ed.). Glenview, IL: Scott Foresman.

Coleman, J. T. (1987). Toward an integrated theory of white-collar crime. *American Journal of Sociology, 93*(2), 406–439.

Coleman, E., Cesnik, J., Moore, A.-M., & Dwyer, M. (1992). An exploratory study of the role of psychotropic medications in the treatment of sex offenders. *Journal of Offender Rehabilitation, 18*(3–4), 75–88.

Columbus Dispatch. (2013). Retrieved November 10, 2016, from http://www.dispatch.com/content/stories/public/2013/08/15/dibble-sentenced.html.

Conrad, S., & Wincze, J. (1976). Orgasmic reconditioning: A controlled study of its effects upon the sexual arousal and behavior of male homosexuals. *Behavior Therapy, 7,* 155–166.

Cox, R. P., & Howard, M. D. (2007). Utilization of EMDR in the treatment of sexual addiction: A case study. *Sexual Addiction and Compulsivity, 14*(1), 1–20.

Cunningham, M. R., Roberts, A. R., Barbee, A. P., & Druen, P. B. (1995). 'Their ideas of beauty are, on the whole, the same as ours': Consistency and variability in the cross-cultural perception of female attractiveness. *Journal of Personality and Social Psychology, 68,* 261–279.

D'Arrigo, A. (2006). *L'Homme Oiseau.* Paris: Arthaud.

Daffern, M., Jones, L., Howells, K., Shine, J., Mikton, C., & Tunbridge, V. (2007). Refining the definition of offence paralleling behaviour. *Criminal Behaviour and Mental Health, 17,* 265–273.

Davidson, P. R., & Parker, C. H. (2001). Eye movement desensitization and reprocessing (EMDR): A meta-analysis. *Journal of Consulting and Clinical Psychology, 69*(2), 305–316.

Dawson, S. J., Bannerman, B. A., & Lalumière, M. (2016). Paraphilic interests: An examination of sex differences in a nonclinical sample. *Sex Abuse: A Journal of Treatment and Research, 28*(1), 20–45.

de Oliveira, W. M., Jr., & Abdo, C. H. N. (2010). Unconventional sexual behaviors and their associations with physical, mental and sexual health parameters: A study in 18 large Brazilian cities. *Revista Brasileira de Psiquiatria, 32*(3), 264–274.

de River, J. P. (1956). *The sexual criminal.* Springfield, IL: Charles C. Thomas.

Delle-Vergini, V., & Day, A. (2016). Case formulation in forensic practice: Challenges and opportunities. *Journal of Forensic Practice, 18*(3), 240–250.

Douglas, J. D., Rasmussen, P. K., & Flanagan, C. A. (1977). *The nude beach.* Beverly Hills, CA: Sage.

Doyle, T. (2009). Privacy and perfect voyeurism. *Ethics and Information Technology, 11,* 181–189.

Duff, S. C. (2010). Exploring criminogenic need through victim apology letters: An interpretative phenomenological analysis. *Journal of Aggression, Conflict and Peace Research, 2*(2), 33–43.

Duff, S. C. (2011). Exploring criminogenic need through victim apology letters II: An IPA analysis of post-treatment accounts of offending against children. *Journal of Aggression, Conflict and Peace Research, 3*(4), 230–242.

Duff, S. C., & Scott, A. J. (2013). Understanding perceptions of stalking: The impact of additional contextual information regarding the breakdown of relationships. *Journal of Criminal Psychology, 3*(2), 136–144.

Eells, T. D. (2007). History and current status of psychotherapy case formulation. In T. D. Eells (Ed.), *Handbook of psychotherapy case formulation* (2nd ed., pp. 3–32). New York: Guilford Press.

Enquist, M., Aronsson, H., Ghirlanda, S., Jansson, L., & Jannini, E. A. (2011). Exposure to mother's pregnancy and lactation in infancy is associated with sexual attraction to pregnancy and lactation in adulthood. *Journal of Sexual Medicine, 8,* 140–147.

Evans, C., Mellor-Clark, J., Margison, F., Barkham, M., Audin, K., Connell, J., & McGrath, G. (2009). CORE: Clinical outcomes in routine evaluation. *Journal of Mental Health, 9*(3), 247–255.

Eysenck, H. J., & Wilson, G. D. (2013). *The experimental study of Freudian theory.* London: Routledge.

Fenichel, O. (1945). *The psychoanalytic theory of neurosis.* New York: Norton.

Fink, B., Hugill, N., & Lange, B. P. (2012). Women's body movements are a potential cue to ovulation. *Personality and Individual Differences, 53*(6), 759–763.

Forsyth, C. J. (1996). The structuring of vicarious sex. *Deviant Behavior, 17*(3), 279–295.

Fox, K. A., Nobles, M. R., & Akers, R. L. (2011). Is stalking a learned phenomenon? An empirical test of social learning theory. *Journal of Criminal Justice, 39*(1), 39–47.

Freud, S. (1938). *Three contributions to the theory of sex.* In The basic writings of Sigmund Freud (pp. 562–563). New York, NY: Random House

Freud, S. (1977). *On sexuality: Three essays on the theory of sexuality and other works.* Harmondsworth: Penguin.

Freund, K. (1988). Courtship disorders: Is this hypothesis valid? *Annals of the New York Academy of Sciences, 528,* 172–182.

Freund, K. (1990). Courtship disorder. In W. L. Marshall, D. R. Laws, & H. E. Barbaree (Eds.), *Handbook of sexual assault: Issues, theories and treatment of the offender* (pp. 195–207). New York: Plenum Press.

Freund, K., Scher, H., Racansky, I. G., Campbell, K., & Heasman, G. (1986). Males disposed to commit rape. *Archives of Sexual Behavior, 15*(1), 23–35.

Freund, K., & Seto, M. C. (1998). Preferential rape in the theory of courtship disorder. *Archives of Sexual Behavior, 27,* 433–443.

Friday, N. (1973). *My Secret Garden: Women's Sexual Fantasies.* NY: Simon and Schuster.

Friday, N. (1975). *Forbidden Flowers: More Women's Sexual Fantasies.* NY: Simon and Schuster.

Friedman, P. (1959). Sexual deviations. In S. Arieti (Ed.), *American handbook of psychiatry* (pp. 589–603). New York: Basic Books.

Furnham, A. (1988). *Lay theories.* Oxford: Pergamon.

Furnham, A. (1989). Overcoming 'psychosomatic' illness: Lay attributions of cure for five possible psychosomattc illnesses. *Social Science and Medicine, 29,* 61–67.

Furnham, A., & Haraldsen, E. (1998). Lay theories of etiology and "cure" for four types of paraphilia: Fetishism; Pedophilia; sexual sadism and voyeurism. *Journal of Clinical Psychology, 54*(5), 689–700.
Furnham, A., & McDermott, M. R. (1994). Lay beliefs about the efficacy of self-reliance, seeking help, and external control as strategies for overcoming obesity, drug addiction, marital problems, stuttering, and insomnia. *Psychology and Health, 9*, 397–406.
Gagnon, J. H., & Simon, W. (2005). *Sexual conduct: The social sources of human sexuality* (2nd ed.). New Brunswick, USA: Aldine Transaction.
Gaupp, L. A., Stern, R. M., & Ratliff, R. G. (1971). The use of aversion-relief procedures in the treatment of a case of voyeurism. *Behavior Therapy, 2*, 585–588.
Gebhard, P. H., Gagnon, J. H., Pomeroy, W. B., & Christenson, C. V. (1965). *Sex offenders*. New York: Harper & Row.
Gelles, R. J. (1983). An exchange/social control theory. In D. Finkelhor, R. J. Gelles, G. Hotaling, & M. A. Straus (Eds.), *The dark side of families* (pp. 182–192). Beverly Hills, CA: Sage.
Gibson, J. J. (1966). *The senses considered as perceptual systems*. Boston: Houghton Mifflin Company.
Gilmour, D. R., McCormick, I. A., & de Ruiter, C. A. (1981). Group assertion training for adult male offenders: Internal validity *Behavior Therapy, 12*, 274–279.
Hammer, E. F. (1968). Symptoms of sexual deviation: Dynamics and etiology. *Psychoanalytic Review, 55*, 5–27.
Harper, D., & Moss, D. (2003). A different kind of chemistry? Reformulating 'formulation'. *Clinical Psychology, 25*, 6–10.
Hawton, K. (1983). Behavioural approaches to the management of sexual deviations. *British Journal of Psychiatry, 143*(3), 248–255.
Heim, N., & Hursch, C. J. (1979). Castration for sexual offenders: Treatment or punishment? A review and critique of recent European literature. *Archives of Sexual Behavior, 8*, 281–304.
Hirschfield, M. (1948). *Sexual anomalies and perversions*. London: Francis Alder.
Ho, S., Foulsham, T., & Kingstone, A. (2015). Speaking and listening with the eyes: Gaze signalling during dyadic interactions. *PLoS One, 10*(8). https://doi.org/10.1371/journal.pone.0136905.
Hocken, K., & Thorne, K. (2012). Voyeurism, exhibitionism and other non-contact sexual offences. In B. Winder & P. Banyard (Eds.), *A psychologist's casebook of crime: From arson to voyeurism*. Houndsmills, UK: Palgrave Macmillan.
Holmes, R. M., Tewksbury, R., & Holmes, S. T. (1998). Hidden JPGs: A functional alternative to voyeurism. *Journal of Popular Culture, 32*(3), 17–29.
Hopkins, T. A., Green, B. A., Carnes, P. J., & Campling, S. (2016). Varieties of intrusion: Exhibitionism and voyeurism. *Sexual Addiction & Compulsivity, 23*(1), 4–33.

Hoyer, J., Kunst, H., & Schmidt, A. (2001). Social phobia as a comorbid condition in sex offenders with paraphilia or impulse control disorder. *The Journal of Nervous and Mental Disease, 189*(7), 463–470.

Husain, W., & Qureshi, Z. (2016). Preferences in marital sexual practices and the role of pornography. *Sexologies, 25,* 35–41.

Jackson, B. T. (1969). A case study of voyeurism treated by counterconditioning. *Behavioral Research & Therapy, 7,* 133–134.

Jones, L. F. (2004). Offence paralleling behaviour (OPB) as a framework for assessment and interventions with offenders. In A. Needs & G. Towl (Eds.), *Applying psychology to forensic practice.* Oxford: Blackwell and British psychological Society.

Jones, B. C., Little, A. C., Burt, D. M., & Perrett, D. I. (2004). When facial attractiveness is only skin deep. *Perception, 33*(5), 569–576.

Joyal, C. C., & Carpentier, J. (2016). The prevalence of paraphilic interests and behaviors in the general population: A provincial survey. *The Journal of Sex Research, 54*(2), 161–171.

Kaplan, M., & Krueger, R. (1997). Voyeurism: Psychopathology and theory. In D. R. Laws & W. O'Donohue (Eds.), *Sexual deviance: Theory, assessment, and treatment* (pp. 297–310). New York, NY: Guilford Press.

Karpman, B. (1954). *The sexual offender and his offences.* New York, NY: Julian Press.

Kendrick, K. M., Hinton, M. R., Atkins, K., Haupt, M. A., & Skinner, J. D. (1998). Mothers determine sexual preferences. *Nature, 395,* 229–230.

Kinderman, P. (2001). The future of clinical psychology training. *Clinical Psychology, 8,* 6–10.

Kleinplatz, P. J. (2014). The paraphilias: An experiential approach to "dangerous" desires. In Y. M. Binik & K. S. K. Hall (Eds.), *Principles and practice of sex therapy* (5th ed., pp. 195–218). New York, NY: Guilford.

Konopacki, W. P., & Oei, T. P. S. (1988). Interruption in the maintenance of compulsive sexual disorder: Two case studies. *Archives of Sexual Behavior, 17,* 411–419.

Koo, K. C., Shim, G. S., Park, H. H., Rha, K. H., Choi, Y. D., Chung, B. H., et al. (2013). Treatment outcomes of chemical castration on Korean sex offenders. *Journal of Forensic and Legal Medicine, 20,* 563–566.

Kutchinsky, B. (1976). Deviance and criminality: The case of voyeur in a peeper's paradise. *Diseases of the Nervous System, 37,* 145–151.

Kuyken, W., Padesky, C. A., & Dudley, R. (2008). The science and practice of case conceptualization. *Behavioural and Cognitive Psychotherapy, 36,* 757–768.

Lamontagne, Y., & Lesage, A. (1986). Private exposure and covert sensitization in the treatment of exhibitionism. *Journal of Behavior Therapy and Experimental Psychiatry, 17,* 197–201.

Landau, S. F., & Freeman-Longo, R. E. (1990). Classifying victims: A proposed multidimensional victimological typology. *International Review of Victimology, 1,* 267–286.

Langevin, R., Paitich, D., & Russon, A. E. (1985). Voyeurism: Does it predict sexual aggression or violence in general? In R. Langevin (Ed.), *Erotic preference, gender identity, and aggression in men: New research studies* (pp. 77–98). Hillsdale, NJ: Erlbaum.

Langlois, J. H., Kalakanis, L., Rubenstein, A. J., Larson, A., Hallam, M., & Smoot, M. (2000). Maxims or myths of beauty? A meta-analytic and theoretical review. *Psychological Bulletin, 126*(3), 390–423.

Långström, N., & Seto, M. C. (2006). Exhibitionistic and voyeuristic behaviour in a Swedish national population sample. *Archives of Sexual Behavior, 35,* 427–435.

Lavin, M. (2008). Voyeurism: Psychopathology and theory. In D. Richard Laws & W. T. O'Donohue (Eds.), *Sexual deviance: Theory, assessment, and treatment* (pp. 305–319). New York, NY: The Guilford Press.

Laws, D. R., & Marshall, W. L. (1990). A conditioning theory of the etiology and maintenance of deviant sexual preference and behavior. In W. L. Marshall & others (Eds.), *Handbook of sexual assault.* New York: Springer Science + Business Media.

Laws, D. R., & Marshall, W. L. (1991). Masturbatory reconditioning of sexual deviates: An evaluative review. *Advances in Behavior Research and Therapy, 13*(1), 13–25.

Leiblum, S. R., & Nathan, S. G. (2001). Persistent sexual arousal syndrome: A newly discovered pattern of female sexuality. *Journal of Sex & Marital Therapy, 27*(4), 365–380.

Leiter, B. (1992). Intellectual voyeurism in legal scholarship. *Yale Journal of the Law and Humanities, 4,* 79–104.

Levy, M. S. (2015). *Celebrity and entertainment obsession: Understanding our addiction.* London: Rowman & Littlefield.

Lewis, A., Grubin, D., Ross, C. C., & Das, M. (2017). Gonadotrophin-releasing hormone agonist treatment for sexual offenders: A systematic review. *Journal of Psychopharmacology, 31*(10), 1281–1293.

Löfgren-Mårtenson, L., & Månsson, S. (2010). Lust, love, and life: A qualitative study of Swedish adolescents' perceptions and experiences with pornography. *Journal of Sex Research, 47,* 568–579.

Longo, R. E., & Groth, A. N. (1983). Juvenile sexual offences in the histories of adult rapists and child molesters. *International Journal of Offender Therapy and Comparative Criminology, 27,* 150–155.

Lorand, S., & Schneer, H. (1967). Sexual deviations. In A. Freedman & H. Kaplan (Eds.), *Comprehensive Textbook of Psychiatry* (pp. 977–988). Baltimore: Williams & Wilkins.

Los Angeles Times. (2015). Retrieved November 10, 2017, from http://www.latimes.com/local/crime/la-me-hollywood-video-voyeur-20150802-story.html.

MacDonald, C., & Mikes-Liu, K. (2009). Is there a place for biopsychosocial formulation in a systemic practice? *The Australian and New Zealand Journal of Family Therapy, 30*(4), 269–283.

Makanjuola, A. B., Adegunloye, O. A., & Adelekan, M. L. (2008). Disorders of sexual preference among secondary school teachers in Ilorin, Nigeria. *Nigerian Journal of Psychiatry, 6*(1), 26–30.

Maletzky, B. M. (1991). *Treating the Sexual Offender.* Thousand Oaks, CA: Sage.

Maletzky, B. M., & McGovern, K. B. (1991). *Treating the sexual offender.* Newbury Park: Sage.

Mann, R. E., Ainsworth, F., Al-Attar, Z., & Davies, M. (2008). Voyeurism: Assessment and treatment. In D. R. Laws & W. T. O'Donohue (Eds.), *Sexual Deviance* (2nd ed., pp. 320–335). New York: Guilford Press.

Margison, F., & Brown, P. (2007). Assessment in psychotherapy. In J. Naismith & S. Grant (Eds.), *Seminars in the Psychotherapies* (pp. 1–27). London: RCPsych Publications.

Marsh, P. J., Odlaug, B. L., Thomarios, N., Davis, A. A., Buchanan, S. N., Meyer, C. S., & Grant, J. E. (2010). Paraphilias in adult psychiatric inpatients. *Annals of Clinical Psychiatry, 22*(2), 129–134.

Marshall, W. L., & Barbaree, H. E. (1978). The reduction of deviant arousal: Satiation treatment for sexual aggressors. *Criminal Justice and Behaviour, 5*(4), 294–303.

Marshall, W. L., & Barbaree, H. E. (1990). An integrated theory of the etiology of sexual offending. In W. L. Marshall, D. R. Laws, & H. E. Barbaree (Eds.), *Handbook of sexual assault: Issues, theories, and treatment of the offender* (pp. 257–271). New York: Springer Science + Business Media.

Marshall, W. L., Fernandez, Y. M., Marshall, L. E., & Serran, G. A. (Eds.). (2006). *Sexual offender treatment: Controversial issues.* Hoboken, NJ: Wiley.

Marshall, W. L., & Williams, S. M. (1975). *A behavioral treatment program for incarcerated sex offenders: Some tentative results.* Paper presented at the Annual Meeting of the Association for the Advancement of Behavior Therapy, San Francisco, December.

Mathews, A., Fox, E., Yiend, J., & Calder, A. (2003). The face of fear: Effects of eye gaze and emotion on visual attention. *Visual Cognition, 10*(7), 823–835.

McAnulty, R. D., Adams, H. E., & Dillon, J. (2001). Sexual deviation: Paraphilias. In P. B. Sutker & H. E. Adams (Eds.), *Comprehensive handbook of psychopathology* (3rd ed., pp. 749–773). New York, NY: Kluwer Academic.

McCloskey, M., & Kohl, D. (1983). Naïve physics: The curvilinear impetus principle and its role in interactions with moving objects. *Journal of Experimental Psychology: Learning, Memory, & Cognition, 9*(1), 146–156.

McConaghy, N. (1970). Subjective and penile plethysmograph responses to aversion therapy for homosexuality: A follow-up study. *British Journal of Psychiatry, 17*, 555–560.

McConaghy, N. (1974). Penile volume responses to moving and still pictures of male and female nudes. *Archives of Sexual Behavior, 3*, 565–570.

McEwan, T. E., Davis, M. R., MacKenzie, R., & Mullen, P. E. (2009). The effects of social desirability response bias on STAXI-2 profiles in a clinical forensic sample. *British Journal of Clinical Psychology, 48,* 431–436.

McGuire, R. J., Carlisle, J. M., & Young, B. G. (1964). Sexual deviations as conditioned behaviour: A hypothesis. *Behavior Research and Therapy, 2*(2–4), 185–190.

Mclatchie, N., Giner-Sorolla, R., & Derbyshire, S. W. G. (2016). 'Imagined guilt' vs 'recollect guilt': Implications for fMRI. *Social and Affective Neuroscience, 11*(5), 703–711.

McNally, M. R., & Fremouw. W. J. (2014). Examining risk of escalation: A critical review of the exhibitionistic behavior literature. *Aggression and Violent Behavior, 19*(5), 474–485.

Mees, H. L. (1966). Sadistic fantasies modified by aversive conditioning and substitution: A case study. *Behaviour Research and Therapy, 4*(4), 317–320.

Money, J. (1986). *Lovemaps: Clinical concepts of sexual/erotic health and pathology, paraphilia, and gender transposition in childhood, adolescence, and maturity.* New York, NY: Irvington.

Morey, L. C. (2007). *The personality assessment inventory professional manual.* Lutz, FL: Psychological Assessment Resources.

Morton, J., & Johnson, M. H. (1991). CONSPEC and CONLERN: A two process theory of infant face recognition. *Psychology Review, 2,* 164–181.

Nelson, A. (1977). A case of voyeurism (scoptophilia). *The Journal of Orgonomy, 11*(1), 57–61.

Nicolosi, A., Laumann, E. O., Glasser, D. B., Moreira, E. D., Jr., Paik, A., & Gingell, C. (2004). Sexual behaviour and sexual dysfunctions after age 40: The global study of sexual attitudes and behaviors. *Adult Urology, 54*(5), 991–997.

Parnell, L. (1999). *EMDR in the treatment of adults abused as children.* New York, NY: Norton.

Pascalis, O., de Schonen, S., Morton, J., Deruelle, C., & Fabre-Grenet, M. (1995). Mother's face recognition by neonates: A replication and an extension. *Infant Behavior Development, 18,* 79–95.

Perry, D. G., & Bussey, K. (1979). The social learning theory of sex differences: Imitation is alive and well. *Journal of Personality and Social Psychology, 37*(10), 1699–1712.

Persons, J. B. (1989). *Cognitive therapy in practice: A case formulation approach.* New York, NY: Norton.

Pinkava, V. (1971). Logical models of sexual deviation. *International Journal of Man-Machine Studies, 3,* 351–374.

Pirelli, B., Esben, E., Almås, E., & Weingarten, K. (2015). Sex positive ways of perceiving sexual turn-on patterns Part I—Understanding. *International Journal of Narrative Therapy & Community Work, 1,* 26–37.

Pound, N. (2002). Male interest in visual cues of sperm competition risk. *Evolution and Human Behavior, 23*(6), 443–466.

Puts, D. A., Bailey, D. H., Cárdenas, R. A., Burriss, R. P., Welling, L. L. M., Wheatley, J. R., & Dawood, K. (2013). Women's attractiveness changes with estradiol and progesterone across the ovulatory cycle. *Hormones and Behavior, 63*(1), 13–19.

Quinn, J. T., Harbisan, J. J., & McAllister, H. (1970). An attempt to shape human penile responses. *Behavior Research and Therapy, 8*, 213–216.

Rachman, S., & Hodgson, R. J. (1968). Experimentally-induced "sexual fetishism": Replication and development. *The Psychological Record, 18*(1), 25–27.

Rangaswamy, K. (1987). Treatment of voyeurism by behavior therapy. *Child Psychiatry Quarterly, 20*, 381–386.

Raven, B. H. (1999). Kurt Lewin address: Influence, power, religion, and the mechanisms of social control. *Journal of Social Issues, 55*(1), 161–186.

Reitz, W. E., & Keil, W. E. (1971). Behavioral treatment of an exhibitionist. *Journal of Behavior Therapy and Experimental Psychiatry, 2*(1), 67–69.

Rhodes, G., Simmons, L. W., & Peters, M. (2005). Attractiveness and sexual behavior: Does attractiveness enhance mating success? *Evolution and Human Behavior, 26*, 186–201.

Rosen, I. (1967). *Pathology and treatment of sexual deviations*. Oxford: Oxford University Press.

Rosen, I. (1979). Exhibitionism, scopophilia and voyeurism. In I. Rosen (Ed.), *Sexual deviation*. Oxford: Oxford University Press.

Rosen, R. C., Shapiro, D., & Schwartz, G. (1975). Voluntary control of penile tumescence. *Psychosomatic Medicine, 37*(6), 479–483.

Rupp, H. A., & Wallen, K. (2007). Sex differences in viewing sexual stimuli: An eye-tracking study in men and women. *Hormones and Behavior, 51*(4), 524–533.

Rye, B. J., & Meaney, G. J. (2007). Voyeurism. *International Journal of Sexual Health, 19*(1), 47–56.

Saleh, F. M., & Berlin, F. (2003). Sex hormones, neurotransmitters, and psychopharmacological treatments in men with paraphilic disorders. *Journal of Child Sexual Abuse, 12*(3–4), 233–253.

Schwartz, B. J. (1956). An empirical test of two Freudian hypotheses concerning castration anxiety. *Journal of Personality, 24*, 318–327.

Serber, M. (1970). Shame aversion therapy. *Journal of Behavioral Therapy and Experimental Psychiatry, 1*, 213–215.

Shapiro, F. (1989). Efficacy of the eye movement desensitization procedure in the treatment of traumatic memories. *Journal of Traumatic Stress, 2*, 199–223.

Shoveller, J. A., Johnson, J. L., Langille, D. B., & Mitchell, T. L. (2004). Socio-cultural influences on young people's sexual behaviour. *Social Science and Medicine, 59*(3), 473–487.

Sidi, H., & Midin, M. (2008). Voyeurism with sexual fantasy on female body parts: A subtype of obsessive-compulsive disorder? *Malaysian Journal of Psychiatry Ejournal, 17*(1), 1–6.

Simon, R. I. (1997). Video voyeurs and the covert videotaping of unsuspecting victims: Psychological and legal consequences. *Journal of Forensic Science, 42*(5), 884–889.

Simpson, P. M., Horton, S., & Brown, G. (1996). Male nudity in advertisements: A modified replication and extension of gender and product effects. *Journal of the Academy of Marketing Science, 24*(3), 257–262.

Singh, D. (1993). Adaptive significance of female physical attractiveness: Role of waist-to-hip ratio. *Journal of Personality and Social Psychology, 65*(2), 293–307.

Singh, D. (1995). Female judgment of male attractiveness and desirability for relationships: Role of waist to-hip ratio and financial status. *Journal of Personality and Social Psychology, 69*(6), 1089–1101.

Slovenko, R. (1965). *Sexual behavior and the law*. Springfield, IL: Charles C. Thomas.

Smith, R. S. (1976). Voyeurism: A literature review. *Archives of Sexual Behavior, 5*(6), 585–608.

Smith, C. A., Ireland, T. O., Park, A., Elwyn, L., & Thornberry, T. P. (2011). Intergenerational continuities and discontinuities in intimate partner violence: A two-generational prospective study. *Journal of Interpersonal Violence, 26*(18), 3720–3752.

Snaith, P. (1983). Exhibitionism: A clinical conundrum. *British Journal of Psychiatry, 143*(3), 231–235.

Sperling, M. (1963). Fetishism in children. *The Psychoanalytic Quarterly, 32*(3), 374–392.

Spielberger, C. (1999). *STAXI-2 state-trait anger expression inventory-2: Professional manual.* Odessa, FL: Psychological Assessment Resources.

Stinson, J. D., & Becker, J. V. (2013). *Treating sex offenders: An evidence-based manual.* New York, NY: The Guildford Press.

Swami, V., Jones, J., Einon, D., & Furnham, A. (2009). Men's preferences for women's profile waist-to-hip ratio, breast size, and ethnic group in Britain and South Africa. *British Journal of Psychology, 100,* 313–325.

Talbot, T. J., & Langdon, P. E. (2006). A revised sexual knowledge assessment tool for people with intellectual disabilities: Is sexual knowledge related to sexual offending behaviour? *Journal of Intellectual Disability Research, 50*(7), 523–531.

Taylor, M., & Quayle, E. (2003). *Child pornography: An Internet crime*. Hove: Brunner-Routledge.

Templeman, T. L., & Stinnett, R. D. (1991). Patterns of sexual arousal and history in a "normal" sample of young men. *Archives of Sexual Behavior, 20,* 137–150.

The Sun. (2017, November 23). Retrieved February 28, 2018, from https://www.thesun.co.uk/news/4970233/man-hid-secret-camera-starbucks-toilet-south-london/.

The Sun. (2018, February 28). Retrieved February 28, 2018, from https://www.thesun.co.uk/news/5682705/randy-couple-romp-in-hotel-room-completely-unaware-that-a-huge-cheering-crowd-is-watching-outside-with-some-even-climbing-up-the-building/.

The Toronto Observer. (2012, October 14). Retrieved February 28, 2018, from https://torontoobserver.ca/2012/10/14/voyeur-websites-under-scrutiny-by-police-and-public/.

Thornhill, R., & Gangestad, S. W. (1999). The scent of symmetry: A human sex pheromone that signals fitness? *Evolution and Human Behavior, 20*(3), 175–201.

Thornhill, R., & Gangestad, S. W. (2006). Facial sexual dimorphism, developmental stability, and susceptibility to disease in men and women. *Evolution and Human Behavior, 27*(2), 131–144.

Thorpe, J. G., Schmidt, E., & Castell, D. (1963). A comparison of positive and negative (aversive) conditioning in the treatment of homosexuality. *Behaviour Research and Therapy, 1*(2–4), 357–362.

Vicedo, M. (2009). The father of ethology and the foster mother of ducks: Konrad Lorenz as an Expert on Motherhood. *Isis, 100*(2), 263–291.

Walton, J. S., & Duff, S. (2017). "I'm not homosexual or heterosexual, I'm paedosexual": Exploring sexual preference for children using interpretive phenomenology. *Journal of Forensic Practice, 19*(2), 151–161.

Wang, E. W., Rogers, R., Giles, C. L., Diamond, P. M., Herrington-Wang, L. E., & Taylor, E. R. (1998). A pilot study of the Personality Assessment Inventory (PAI) in corrections: Assessment of malingering, suicide risk, and aggression in male inmates. *Behavioral Sciences & the Law, 15*(4), 469–482.

Weinberg, M. S., Williams, C. J., & Calhan, C. (1995). "If the shoe fits…": Exploring male homosexual foot fetishism. *The Journal of Sex Research, 32*(1), 17–27.

Wernik, U. (1993). The role of traumatic component in the etiology of sexual dysfunctions and its treatment with eye movement desensitization procedure. *Journal of Sex Education and Therapy, 19*, 212–222.

Wickramasekera, I. (1972). A technique for controlling a certain type of sexual exhibitionism. *Psychotherapy: Theory, Research and Practice, 9*(3), 207–210.

Woodson, J. C. (2002). Including 'learned sexuality' in the organization of sexual behaviour. *Neuroscience and Biobehavioral Reviews, 26*, 69–80.

Wynn, C., & Duff, S. (2016). *Offence Patterns in Repeat Sexual Offenders: An examination of escalation, de-escalation, and stability across sexual offence categories.* Division of Forensic Psychology Annual Conference, Manchester Metropolitan University, England, June 2016.

Yalom, I. D. (1960). Aggression and forbiddenness in voyeurism. *Archives of General Psychiatry, 3*(3), 305–319.

YouGov. (2016). *The last days of the Y Front.* https://yougov.co.uk/news/2016/08/12/exposed-britains-underwear-preferences-unveiled/.

Index

S. Duff, *Voyeurism*, https://doi.org/10.1007/978-3-319-97160-5